Medical Library

Queen's University Belfast
Tel: 028 9063 2500
E-mail: med.issue@qub.ac.uk

For due dates and renewals:

QUB borrowers see 'MY ACCOUNT' at
http://library.qub.ac.uk/qcat
or go to the Library Home Page

HPSS borrowers see 'MY ACCOUNT' at
www.honni.qub.ac.uk/qcat

This book must be returned not later
than its due date but may be recalled
earlier if in demand

Fines are imposed on overdue books

An Illustrated Guide to
Dental Care for the Medically Compromised Patient

Margaret C. Grundy
L.D.S., F.D.S.R.C.S., D.D.S.
Formerly Senior Lecturer and Honorary Consultant
Birmingham Dental School

Linda Shaw
B.D.S., PhD., F.D.S.R.C.S.
Senior Lecturer and Honorary Consultant
Birmingham Dental School

David V. Hamilton
M.A., M.B., B.Chir., F.R.C.P.
Consultant Physician
Norfolk and Norwich Hospital

Wolfe Publishing

Copyright © 1993 Mosby–Year Book Europe Limited
Published in 1993 by Wolfe Publishing, an imprint of
Mosby–Year Book Europe Limited
Printed by BPCC Hazells Ltd., Aylesbury, England.
ISBN 0 7234 1707 5

A CIP catalogue record for this book is available from the British Library.

For full details of all Mosby–Year Book Europe Limited titles please
write to Mosby–Year Book Europe Limited, Brook House, 2–16
Torrington Place, London WC1E 7LT, England.

Contents

Preface

The aim of this book is to provide information to enable the dentist to understand better the more common conditions that will be met with in the care of those people who are medically compromised and may have special needs. We also include those conditions that, by their rarity, should be recognisable as requiring special attention.

The medical management is included and also, where applicable, the appropriate modifications for dental treatment.

Although efforts have been made to cover all age groups there is a paediatric slant in our writing and illustrations, as many of the conditions described are first apparent in the child patient.

Traditionally, paediatric dentists have been mainly responsible for the dental care of those with special needs. This has perhaps been particularly appropriate for those with learning difficulties as the philosophy of their management has been similar to that for children.

Most dental schools now include some teaching about the care of those with special needs, but only a limited time is available in the curriculum. In recent years, with the emphasis on 'normalisation' and care in the community, many people who are medically compromised and who may have special needs will seek treatment from a general dental practitioner.

In the past, dentists were reluctant to accept these patients because of a feeling of inadequacy. Knowledge of their condition helps the dentist to overcome these fears; this book will contribute towards this aim, and thus improve the care of these disadvantaged people.

Although written with dentists in mind, we feel that dental undergraduates, postgraduate students, hygienist students, hygienists and, in fact, all who provide dental care for this special group of people, will benefit from the information herein.

Acknowledgements

Most of the illustrations are of our own patients and we are grateful to them for giving us permission to use their pictures. Additional material has been provided by Professor T.D. Foster, Mr John Hamburger, Dr A.S.T. Franks, and Dr J. Leslie. We would also like to thank Miss S. Davenport for **14, 16** and **19**. We are grateful to Churchill Livingstone for giving us permission to use **1–7** and **90** previously published in *Principles of Pathology for Dental Students* by Walter, Hamilton and Israel. We are also grateful to Wolfe Publishing Ltd for allowing us to use a number of pictures previously published in *Diagnostic Picture Tests in Paediatric Dentistry*, by Rock, Grundy and Shaw and also pictures from *A Colour Atlas of Aids,* by Farthing, Brown and Staughton. *Dental Update* have also given permission for the use of **20, 74**, and **122**, which were published in articles by Grundy and Shaw.

The photographic departments of our various hospitals are to be commended for the high standard of the illustrations.

Introduction

With the recent advances in medicine over the past two decades, many children who would have died in infancy are now living into adult age. At the other end of the spectrum, there is a rapidly growing number of people with a greatly increased life span.

Recent data from the United Kingdom show that 18% of the population is over the age of retirement, and there is an increasing proportion who are over 70 years of age. This reflects in a greater prevalence of long-term illness and disability and also of the more complex dental problems experienced in old age.

It is therefore important that dental surgeons and others concerned with the care of those people who are medically compromised are aware of their special needs and problems. This group includes those with physically handicapping conditions, those with learning difficulties, and those who are medically compromised.

The severity of such problems varies from a minor abnormality to a severe impairment resulting in total dependency. An important aspect, however, is the individual response to the impairment. As far as dentistry is concerned, people are only handicapped if they are unable to obtain dental treatment in the ordinary way. However, there are also various medical conditions in which general health may be put at risk further if there is dental disease or when invasive dental treatment is necessary. Moreover, the dentist must be aware of potential complications whilst undertaking routine dental care.

A comprehensive medical history must be obtained so that an assessment may be made regarding the general health of those seeking dental care. It is necessary to know whether the patient is attending or receiving treatment from a doctor, specialist, clinic or hospital, and if the patient is taking any pills, tablets, medicines, tonics or injections. If in doubt about their medication, patients should be asked to bring their medicines with them when attending for treatment.

It may be necessary to communicate with any medical colleague who is also treating the patient. Enquiries about known allergies, particularly antibiotics, are essential as it is indefensible, as well as life threatening, to prescribe medication to which the patient has previously exhibited an allergic response (*see* page 25).

Many elderly people suffer a large number of diseases and disabilities for which different drugs are prescribed. Around one in five of all elderly people take three or more different tablets daily, and one in ten takes four or more medicines daily.

1 Cardiovascular Disorders

There is a wide range of conditions that affect the heart and blood vessels. These cardiovascular disorders can be divided into two main groups, those that are congenital (existing before or at birth – literally 'born with', although their manifestations may not be present for some years after birth), and those which are acquired (developing after birth).

Congenital Heart Defects

There is a wide range of cardiac abnormalities with many variations. Some defects are so slight as to cause no disability and may only be discovered at a routine medical examination. With more severe defects, the child may be breathless on exertion, tire easily, and suffer from recurrent respiratory infections. With very severe defects, the child may be cyanotic, have stunted growth and fail to thrive. Malformations, if sufficiently severe, impose a strain on the ventricle which may lead to myocardial hypertrophy and add to the load already placed on the heart by the primary lesion.

The incidence of congenital heart disease varies among clinical studies, but probably is about 1% of live births. A significant proportion of babies die within the first few weeks of life and a similar number before their first birthday. The outlook has improved in recent years with the development and advancement of surgical and anaesthetic techniques. Recently, cardiac transplantation has been performed on babies only days old with severe life threatening cardiac conditions but as yet the long-term prognosis for these children is not known.

Congenital abnormalities may be divided into four groups:

- Incompatible with fetal survival.
- Compatible with fetal survival, but not with independent neonatal existence.
- Succumb before 2 years of age.
- Survive childhood and may reach adult life. In these:
  (a) cardiac function may be seriously impaired;
  (b) no functional incapacity at rest but at risk when the heart is stressed; and
  (c) no functional disability, but at risk of bacterial endocarditis.

Alternatively, they may be classified more simply as cyanotic or non-cyanotic.

The aetiology is rarely known and may be genetic or environmental. Chromosomal abnormalities, such as Down's syndrome (*see* pages 65–67), only account for a small percentage of cases. The heart forms during weeks 3–8 of intrauterine life, so that certain maternal infections during the first trimester may result in malformations. This is at a time when the woman may be unaware of her pregnancy. Rubella (German measles, *see* page 105) is known to affect the developing heart, and measles, mumps and cytomegalovirus have also been implicated. Women on anticonvulsant drugs, such as phenytoin may also produce babies with heart defects (*see* page 78). However, if the drugs are discontinued during pregnancy, the resultant epileptic fits may also have an undesirable effect on the developing fetus as a result of hypoxia.

Heart murmurs

Heart murmurs may only be discovered at a routine medical examination. They occur in about 75% of children, are caused by turbulence in blood flow and are usually benign and disappear in late childhood. However, murmurs may indicate the presence of a cardiac lesion. If in doubt, cardiological opinion should be obtained.

Patent ductus arteriosus

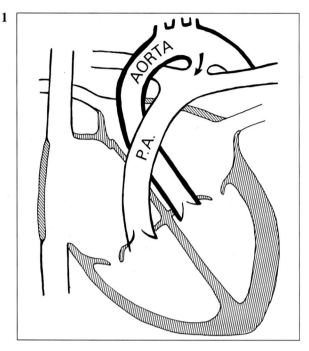

1 Patent ductus arteriosus (courtesy of Churchill Livingstone).

Before birth, in patent ductus arteriosus (**1**) the pressure in the aorta and the pulmonary artery are approximately equal, the lungs are non-functional, and the ductus arteriosus allows the fetal circulation to bypass the lungs. At birth, when the baby starts to breathe, the pressure falls in the pulmonary artery and rises in the aorta. If the embryonic ductus arteriosus fails to close, blood passes from the aorta to the pulmonary artery, thus increasing the volume of blood passing through the lungs and returning to the left atrium and ventricle.

Medical management

Surgical closure by ligation may be required, but indo-methacin, a prostaglandin synthetase inhibitor, may achieve closure in some infants.

Dental care

There seems to be some controversy regarding prophylactic antibiotic therapy for certain dental procedures. Most children may be considered to have normal hearts following corrective surgery, and require prophylactic antibiotics for only the initial 6 months following surgery. A small number of patients may have some recurrent patency following surgery and may be at risk of bacterial endocarditis. The paediatrician should be consulted regarding antibiotic prophylaxis (*see* the recommendations for endocarditis prophylaxis, pages 19, 20).

Ventricular septal defect

Ventricular septal defect (2), a common cardiac malformation, probably accounts for 25% of all congenital heart defects. There is a shunt of oxygenated blood through the defect causing the same changes in the heart and pulmonary blood flow as in patent ductus arteriosus.

Medical management

Many small defects are symptomless and a number close spontaneously during the first few years of life. Large defects require early surgery to save the child's life. In others there may be a reduced exercise tolerance, a tendency to respiratory infections and failure to thrive.

Dental care

Antibiotic prophylaxis is necessary for invasive dental treatment, that is treatment which may result in a bacteraemia; scaling the teeth, sub-gingival restorations, extractions or any treatment procedure which breeches the skin or mucous membranes (*see* pages 19, 20).

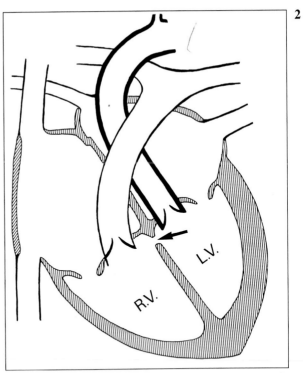

2

2 Ventricular septal defect (courtesy of Churchill Livingstone).

Atrial septal defect

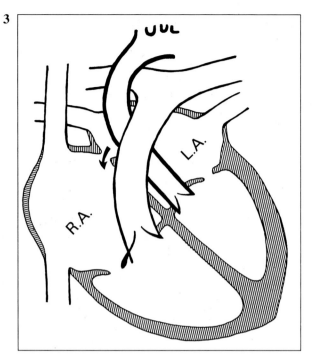

Atrial septal defect (**3**) is the most common congenital defect found in adults and occurs more frequently in females. There is a left-to-right shunt which results in overfilling of the right atrium, right ventricle and pulmonary artery. Children with this lesion tire easily and suffer from frequent respiratory infections.

Medical management

Surgery is advisable before school age. If the condition is not treated cardiac failure may occur in the third decade and life expectancy is reduced.

Dental care

Antibiotic prophylaxis is necessary for invasive dental treatment (*see* pages 19, 20).

3 Atrial septal defect (courtesy of Churchill Livingstone).

Aortic stenosis

Aortic stenosis (**4**) accounts for about 5% of congenital heart abnormalities in children and occurs more frequently in boys than girls. It is also an important cause of cardiac disability in elderly males, although it may occur at any time. It is more commonly due to abnormalities of the valves, when the cusps, usually two instead of three, are partly adherent and frequently malformed. There is obstruction of the blood flow from the left ventricle, which results in ventricular hypertrophy. Exercise tolerance is low and sudden death may occur following exertion. Competitive sports are contraindicated. A congenital bicuspid valve may occur and may be asymptomatic unless it becomes calcified or affected by endocarditis.

Medical management

Surgical treatment is important before ventricular hypertrophy develops. Recent advances with balloon dilatation are now also being used, thereby avoiding surgery in some patients.

Dental care

Prophylactic antibiotics (*see* pages 19, 20) are necessary in order to avoid endocarditis, and there may be a risk with general anaesthesia.

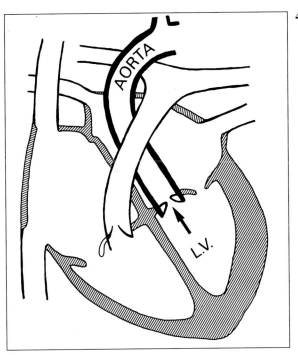

4 Aortic stenosis (courtesy of Churchill Livingstone).

Pulmonary stenosis

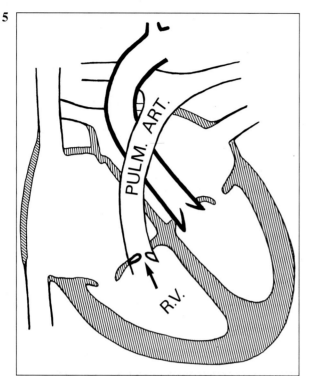

In pulmonary stenosis (**5**) the valves are malformed, resulting in hypertrophy of the right ventricle and eventual cardiac failure. Severe stenosis may result in death in infancy.

Medical management

Balloon dilatation is reported to give good results.

Dental care

If the condition is mild and treatment was not thought necessary to correct the stenosis, then antibiotic cover probably is not required. However, those who have had operative intervention are susceptible to endocarditis and may also be at risk with general anaesthesia.

5 Pulmonary stenosis (courtesy of Churchill Livingstone).

Coarctation of the aorta

In coarctation of the aorta (**6**) there is constriction or narrowing of the aorta, and this usually occurs at about the origin of the ductus arteriosus, just below the origin of the subclavian artery. The blood pressure is raised in the upper part of the body and lowered in the lower extremities: this is usually diagnostic.

Medical management

Resection of the narrowed area is necessary in the first 2 years of life. Untreated patients are likely to die in their thirties from bacterial endocarditis, subarachnoid haemorrhage or hypertensive heart failure.

Dental care

Bacterial endocarditis may develop at the site of the coarctation and prophylactic antibiotics are therefore necessary in patients whether or not they have had surgery.

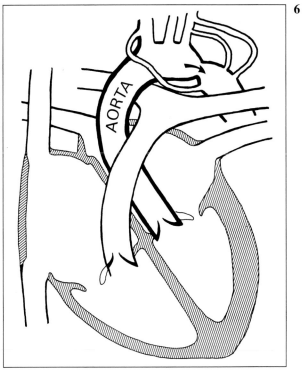

6 Coarctation of the aorta (courtesy of Churchill Livingstone).

Fallot's tetralogy

Fallot's tetralogy (**7**) consists of the combination of:

- Pulmonary stenosis.
- Ventricular septal defect.
- Dextro-position of the aorta.
- Right ventricular hypertrophy.

At first, cyanosis may occur only during crying or feeding, but it usually becomes progressive and persistent as the child gets older. The child has a dusky appearance (**8**) all tissues appear bluish in colour, including the mucous membrane of the lips and tongue (**9, 10**). Dyspnoea occurs with exertion and the child characteristically assumes a squatting position. It is believed that the squatting position, by compressing the abdominal aorta and the femoral arteries, increases the arterial resistance and therefore diminishes the right to left shunt. Clubbing of the fingers and toes is quite common. Growth and development are delayed.

7

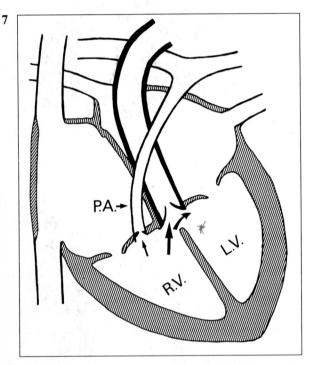

8

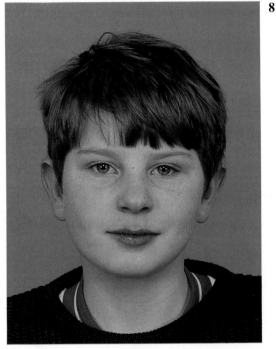

7 Fallot's tetralogy (courtesy of Churchill Livingstone).

8 This boy has Fallot's tetralogy. He has marked cyanosis and delayed growth and development.

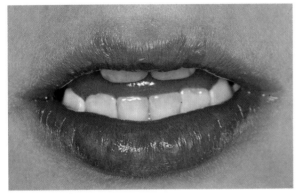

9 Cyanosis affecting the lips in the boy shown in **8**.

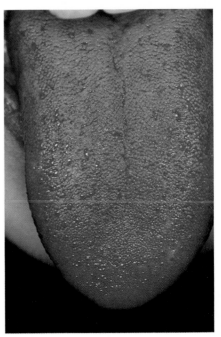

10 Central cyanosis affecting the tongue of the boy shown in **8**.

Medical management

Surgery may be necessary at an early stage in life and consists of relief of obstruction from the right ventricle and closure of the ventricular septal defect (**11**).

Dental care

Antibiotic cover is necessary for dental procedures that are likely to produce a bacteraemia. General anaesthesia is hazardous and may be life threatening.

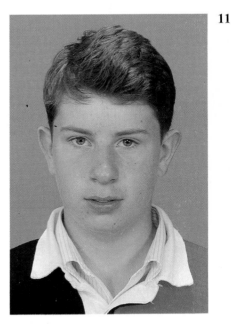

11 Boy shown in **8** two years after major cardiac surgery. Cyanosis is no longer present and considerable growth has occurred.

Marfan's syndrome (arachnodactyly)

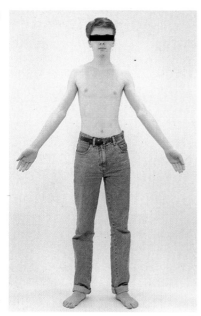

12 A 14-year-old boy with Marfan's syndrome who is above average height and has an increased arm span.

This syndrome, described by Marfan in 1896, is an autosomal dominant disorder of connective tissue. It is included in this section as the principal defect is that of aortic incompetence and dissecting aneurysm which occurs as a result of necrosis of the media of the aorta. The other manifestations are ocular and skeletal. These patients are taller than normal, have an excessively long arm span and long thin spidery fingers (**12**), hence the name arachnodactyly. There is hyperextensibility of the joints and scoliosis (curvature of the spine), and a high arched palate. There may be subluxation or dislocation of the lens and there may be spontaneous detachment of the retina. Cystic disease of the lungs and spontaneous pneumothorax can also occur.

Medical management

This involves correction of ocular defects. In girls, the induction of puberty at the age of 10 years may reduce the ultimate height by early closure of the epiphysis. The scoliosis may require orthopaedic surgical correction.

There has been some success in managing the problem of aortic aneurysm, which is usually the cause of death, by replacement of the ascending aorta.

Dental care

There may be problems with wound healing due to the defective connective tissue, and suturing should be avoided. General anaesthesia may prove hazardous in these patients.

Acquired Cardiovascular Disease

Rheumatic fever

Rheumatic fever is a systemic disease following a Lancefield's Group A streptococcal infection of the upper respiratory tract and involves the joints and the heart. Children aged 5–15 years used to be susceptible in the Western World, now with better standards of living this is extremely rare. The use of antibiotics and the early treatment of streptococcal upper respiratory tract infections may also be a factor.

Rheumatic fever is still a major problem in developing countries, and rheumatic heart disease is the most common form of heart disease in older children and young adults. It is also the main cause of death from heart disease in those over the age of 45 years. The difference seems to be due to the poor socio-economic conditions, overcrowding and poor living conditions, prevalent in the developing countries, and lack of antibiotics.

There is usually a history of a sore throat 2 or 3 weeks previously. There is an immune-complex mediated reaction between the streptococcal antigen and antibody produced by the patient. The soluble antigen–antibody complexes are deposited in the small blood vessels of the heart and joints, and by activating complement lead to tissue damage. The child has a high temperature and is acutely ill. There is pain in the joints (arthralgia), and inflammation (arthritis) with swelling, redness and heat. The lower limbs are particularly affected, usually the knees and ankles. There appears to be a 'flitting pain' from one joint to another. The heart is affected in about 40–50% of patients. The valves become swollen and where the valve cusps meet there are depositions of thrombi on the endocardial surface. These depositions appear as small nodules along the valve closure. Changes may be detected on an electrocardiogram .

Most lesions undergo resolution, but not those on the valves. The cusps become thickened, fibrosed and contracted, with resultant stenosis and/or regurgitation.

Medical management

Bed rest for about 3 weeks is necessary during the acute phase in order to reduce the work of the heart. Antibiotics are given to eradicate infection and salicylates are given to reduce fever and joint pain. Corticosteroids are effective and may be used to relieve the acute exudative phase.

Dental care

Antibiotic prophylaxis is necessary for invasive dental treatment in all patients who have a history of rheumatic fever (*see* pages 19, 20).

Infective endocarditis

Infective endocarditis is an inflammation of the endothelial lining of the heart and may be secondary to bacterial, fungal, or, more rarely, rickettsial infection. The organisms tend to settle on damaged endocardial surfaces, but predominantly on valves which are congenitally deformed or damaged by previous disease.

Although, not proven that antibiotics prevent infective endocarditis in those people with significant cardiac defects, it is generally accepted that prophylactic antibiotics should be given prior to extractions, scaling or other invasive treatments or during procedures which may cause a bacteraemia (for example instrumentation or surgery of the alimentary or genito–urinary tract). However, endocarditis occurs in about 50% of patients without known cardiac defects, e.g. bicuspid aortic valves. The usual organisms are *Streptococcus viridans* (50%) and *Streptococcus faecalis* (10%).

There are approximately 1,400 cases a year in the UK resulting in around 200 deaths annually, 0.1% of all cardiac deaths. About 25% of those affected have a history of congenital heart disease, 25% have had rheumatic heart disease and 25% have had calcific aortic disease, with unknown causes accounting for the remaining 25%. A history of previous dental treatment has been recorded in 10–30% of patients and some dental surgeons have been uncertain about compliance with recommendations. Recent reports have shown that only about three-quarters of dentists are following current guidelines.

The onset may be insidious with weakness, weight loss, tiredness, fever, night sweats and anorexia. Urinalysis reveals haematuria, and apart from the cardiac lesion there may also be enlargement of the spleen. The characteristic appearance of haemorrhages under the nails has led to the descriptive term of splinter haemorrhages (**13**).

Diagnosis is confirmed by the identification of organisms in a blood culture, but treatment is commenced without waiting for the result.

13 Splinter haemorrhages under the nails in a patient with bacterial endocarditis.

Medical management

Early active treatment with high levels of antibiotics is necessary (after blood has been taken for culture), and this may need to be sustained for about 4–6 weeks, depending on the organism and its sensitivity. Of those patients who survive bacterial endocarditis, 20% may have some incapacity caused by complications and many of them will subsequently require surgery to replace damaged valves.

Dental care

The aim of dental care is the prevention of infective endocarditis in susceptible patients, firstly by preventing dental disease but, if treatment is required, by administering the appropriate antibiotics and thus reducing the possibility of even a transient bacteraemia. Scaling the teeth or even periodontal probing may give rise to a bacteraemia.

Endodontics in permanent anterior teeth with mature

apices is probably acceptable provided that treatment is carried out under antibiotic cover and a good apical seal is obtained. Proven endocarditis following endodontic treatment is extremely rare. However, pulp therapy in primary teeth may result in a potential area of infection and therefore should not be carried out.

It has been suggested that all patients should be given antibiotic cover for invasive and manipulative procedures including all dental care. However, if this procedure were to be followed probably more patients would die as a result of anaphylaxis than from endocarditis (*see* page 25).

There is no necessity to give antibiotics for restorative treatment that does not involve the gingiva. If there are positive signs of heart disease and a general anaesthetic is required, the patient should be treated in hospital for this procedure.

The necessity of regular dental care and the maintenance of good oral health should be emphasised to all patients who may be at risk. An application of an antiseptic, such as 0.2% chlorhexidine gluconate, to the gingival margin before dental treatment supplements the antibiotics. Prior to cardiac surgery all patients should be screened for dental disease and made dentally fit and any doubtful teeth extracted.

Prosthetic valve endocarditis

There have been major advances in prosthetic valve replacement, using either a porcine xenograft or a mechanical ball and cage. These valves may last for 10–15 years but require regular follow-up for life.

Prosthetic valve endocarditis (PVE), although uncommon, is life threatening, and may occur within a few months of valve replacement or subsequently as a result of dental treatment or urological procedures.

Medical management

If PVE is suspected, early antibiotic therapy should be commenced after taking a blood sample for culture. Initially, intravenous antibiotics are necessary for a period of 2 weeks, followed by oral antibiotics for up to 2 months.

Dental care

Patients who have prosthetic valves require antibiotic cover for all invasive procedures, as recommended below.

Antibiotic prophylaxis of infective endocarditis

For dental extractions, scaling, or periodontal surgery there are three categories: local anaesthesia, general anaesthesia, and special risk patients.

Under local anaesthesia

For patients not allergic to penicillin and not prescribed penicillin more than once in the previous month, use amoxycillin:

- Adults: 3g single oral dose taken under supervision 1 hour before dental procedures.
- Children under 10: half adult dose.
- Children under 5: quarter adult dose.

For patients allergic to penicillin use either erythromycin stearate:

- Adults: 1.5g orally taken under supervision 1–2 hours before dental procedure plus 0.5g 6 hours later.
- Children under 10: half adult dose.
- Children under 5: quarter adult dose.

or clindamycin:

- Adults: 600mg single oral dose taken under supervision 1 hour before dental procedure.
- Children under 10: 6 mg/kg body weight single oral dose taken under supervision 1 hour before dental procedure.

Under general anaesthesia

For patients not allergic to penicillin and not prescribed penicillin more than once in the previous month use either amoxycillin intramuscularly:

- Adults 1g in 2.5ml 1% lignocaine hydrochloride just before induction plus 0.5g by mouth 6 hours later.
- Children under 10: half adult dose.

or amoxycillin orally:

- Adults 3g oral dose 4 hours before anaesthesia followed by a further 3g by mouth as soon as possible after the operation.
- Children under 10: half adult dose.
- Children under 5: quarter adult dose.

or amoxycillin and probenecid orally:

- Adults: amoxycillin 3g together with probenecid 1g orally 4 hours before the operation.

Special risk patients who should be referred to hospital

Such patients include:

- Patients with prosthetic valves who are to have a general anaesthetic.
- Patients who are to have a general anaesthetic and who are allergic to penicillin or have had penicillin more than once in the previous month.
- Patients who have had a previous attack of endocarditis.

Recommendations for patients not allergic to penicillin and who have not had penicillin more than once in the previous month are:

- Adults: 1g amoxycillin intramuscularly in 2.5ml 1% lignocaine hydrochloride plus 120 mg gentamicin intramuscularly just before induction: then 0.5g amoxycillin orally 6 hours later.
- Children under 10: amoxycillin, half adult dose; gentamicin 2 mg/kg body weight.

Recommendations for patients allergic to penicillin or who have had penicillin more than once in the previous month are:

- Adults: vancomycin 1g by slow intravenous infusion over 60 minutes followed by gentamicin 120mg intravenously just before induction or 15 minutes before surgical procedure.
- Children under 10: vancomycin 20mg /kg intravenously, gentamicin 2mg /kg intravenously.

For further information, see:

- Recommendations from the Endocarditis Working Party of the British Society for Antimicrobial Chemotherapy (1990), *Lancet,* **355**, 88–89.
- Gould, I.M. (1990), Current prophylaxis for the prevention of infective endocarditis, *Br. Dental J.,* **168**, 409–410.

Coronary artery disease (ischaemic heart disease)

Coronary artery disease is a leading cause of death in the UK in men over the age of 40 years and in women over the age of 50 years. It is commonly caused by atherosclerosis which is due to fatty deposits and fibrous plaques in the walls of the coronary arteries.

The specific cause is unknown, however a number of factors increase the risk. Although the condition occurs world-wide, the incidence appears to be higher in certain countries; the reasons for this are not fully understood.

There is some evidence to show that hereditary factors play a part, as there appears to be a greater risk of developing coronary artery disease in those individuals who have had parents or siblings affected before the age of 55 years.

There is an increased incidence in smokers, the greater the number of cigarettes smoked the higher the risk. Moreover, the increased risk may persist, although decrease in time, in those who have given up smoking. Indeed, it is not for 20 years that the risk of heart disease in former smokers equates with non-smokers. Alcoholics and 'heavy drinkers' also have an increased incidence. However non-drinkers have a higher incidence than those who drink a moderate amount of alcohol (less than 14 units/week for women and less than 21 units/week for men). The protective effect of alcohol appears to relate to wine and not spirits.

Possibly the greatest risk of coronary arteriosclerosis is related to hypercholesterolaemia and to low levels of high-density lipoprotein (HDL) cholesterol which is cardioprotective. Other risk factors include hypertension, diabetes and stressful events.

The lumina of the arteries are reduced resulting in deprivation of oxygen to the myocardium. The process begins in childhood with areas of diffuse thickening in the walls of the arteries which are particularly apparent at the bifurcation of the vessels. Angina pectoris may be the first symptom of coronary artery disease. Pain, which is crushing or constricting in nature, is experienced in the substernal region and may radiate across the chest into the arms, neck or up into the jaw. Occasionally this may be mistaken for toothache, but the pain in the jaw recedes with rest.

One can do no better than refer to William Heberden's description of angina in 1768:

'There is a disorder of the breast, marked with strong and peculiar symptoms considerable for the kind of danger belonging to it, and not extremely rare, of which I do not recollect any mention among medical authors. The seat of it, and sense of strangling and anxiety of which it is attended may make it not improperly be called angina pectoris. Those, who are afflicted with it, are seized, while they are walking, and more particularly when they walk soon after eating, with a painful and disagreeable sensation in the breast, which seems as if it would take their life away, if it were to increase or continue: the moment they stand still, all this uneasiness vanishes.'

Angina may be experienced when more demand is placed on the heart, such as in exercise or stress, and usually abates in 10–15 minutes. Failure to resolve in this period may indicate permanent damage from myocardial infarction.

Myocardial infarction is characterised by a discomfort or pain, similar to angina, but lasting for more than 15 minutes. The patient may have a rapid pulse rate, raised or lowered blood pressure and look pale: the pain from myocardial infarction is often more severe than angina and may indeed last for several hours.

Medical management

Glyceryl trinitrate has been the drug of choice for acute relief of ischaemic heart disease for many years, either placed sublingually or sprayed on the buccal mucosa. It causes arterial and venous dilatation, thus reducing the workload of the heart. Although effective, its use may be restricted as it may induce the development of headaches. Beta-blocking agents or calcium antagonists, such as nifedipine, are commonly used for prophylaxis as well as oral nitrates.

In recent years, much success has been achieved by surgical techniques to bypass the coronary artery stenosis by using a vein. The long saphenous vein of the leg is used and post-operative problems are mainly related to the leg. Furthermore, balloon dilatation (percutaneous transluminal angioplasty) may be employed in those considered unfit, because of co-existing disease, for surgery.

Dental care

Patients with a history of myocardial infarction within the previous 6 months should not receive routine dental care. Sudden death, although rare, may occur in the dental chair.

In those with known coronary artery disease, effective local anaesthesia is absolutely essential for treatment in order to avoid endogenous release of adrenaline as a result of painful stimuli. There has been controversy regarding the use of adrenaline as a vasoconstrictor in the local anaesthetic solution for patients with cardiovascular disease. The adrenaline in the local anaesthetic results in more prolonged anaesthesia and may be used unless only a short procedure is planned when it is unnecessary. An alternative vasoconstrictor, felypressin, in conjunction with prilocaine hydrochloride may be used. There should be no problem in those people with mild or moderate cardiovascular disease but vasoconstrictors should be avoided in those with poorly controlled coronary artery disease.

An aspirating syringe must be used in order to avoid intravascular injection and the anaesthetic solution should be administered slowly. If myocardial infarction occurs the treatment is to administer oxygen and give appropriate analgesics (morphine 4–6mg intravenously), the patient should then be transferred to hospital.

Cardiac arrhythmias

Cardiac arrhythmias are any variation from the normal rhythm of the heart. They may occur in normal healthy people and be of little consequence. Conversely, they may produce symptoms which may be of significance to the dentist and may actually be life threatening.

Pacemakers

The first pacemakers were implanted into hearts in 1959. Now over 200,000 are fitted world-wide each year with remarkable success. They are used in the management of abnormalities in the conductive system of the heart. The pacing system consists of a generator which produces a small electric impulse that is transmitted by a lead to an electrode that is in contact with endocardial or myocardial tissue.

Dental care

With the large number of pacemakers which are being fitted annually, it is important that the dentist is aware if the patient has a pacemaker in order to avoid unnecessary problems. Electromagnetic interference from non-cardiac electrical signals may interfere with those of the pacemaker. Certain pulp testers, cavitron scalers, diathermy and electrocautery may all cause problems and should *not* be used.

Heart failure

Heart failure occurs as a result of the inability of the myocardium of the left and/or the right ventricle to contract adequately in such a way that the cardiac output is insufficient for the needs of the body. In left heart failure there is congestion of the pulmonary circulation, leading to dyspnoea, and there may be inadequate tissue perfusion, resulting in fatigue. Right heart failure is commonly associated with left heart failure and results in systemic venous hypertension and peripheral oedema.

Left heart failure

This occurs predominantly in association with progressive damage to the left ventricle secondary to hypertension, aortic stenosis, mitral valve disease, a large ventricular septal defect, or more acutely, as a result of myocardial infarction. As a consequence of pulmonary congestion there is a varying severity of dyspnoea. There may only be mild dyspnoea which occurs on effort, to 'pulmonary oedema' with severe dyspnoea, tachypnoea, sweating, hypoxia, cyanosis and severe anxiety.

Medical management

Mild heart failure may be treated with diuretics, angiotensin converting enzyme inhibitors (ACEI) and control of any arrhythmia (particularly atrial fibrillation) which may have precipitated the failure.

Pulmonary oedema requires urgent treatment. The patient should be sat up (not placed supine), oxygen administered, diuretics given intravenously and diamorphine administered. The diamorphine not only relieves the anxiety but results in some vasodilatation and thus reduces the work of the heart.

In some patients with severe heart failure wheezing may occur (cardiac asthma) which may, by the inexperienced, be mistaken for bronchial asthma.

Dental care

Patients with incipient heart failure should not be treated in the supine position and if a general anaesthetic is required, careful pre-operative assessment is mandatory.

Right heart failure

This usually occurs secondary to left ventricular failure, but may occur *de novo* as a consequence of acute lung disease, for example a large pulmonary embolism or, more commonly, as a result of chronic lung disease (cor pulmonale) from chronic obstructive airways disease. As a result of the elevated right atrial pressure, congestion occurs backward in the circulation, resulting in hepatomegaly (enlargement of the liver) and dependent pitting oedema.

Marked pitting ankle oedema may be due to other causes, for example peripheral venous insufficiency, deep vein thrombosis, and hypoproteinaemia from whatever cause. The dentist should be alerted to the possibility of heart failure and the patient referred for further investigation.

Medical management

Right heart failure may be relieved if the cause is treated, although diuretics may also be required.

Hypertension

Hypertension may be defined as an elevated blood pressure, either systolic or diastolic, above the average blood pressure for the age of the individual. In general, a systolic pressure greater than 160mmHg and a diastolic pressure greater than 90–95mmHg is considered elevated. However, the age of the patient should be taken into account as blood pressure tends to rise with age.

Hypertension is but one of the risk factors for cerebrovascular and cardiovascular disease (both ischaemic heart and peripheral vascular disease) as well as contributing to the development of chronic renal failure.

Hypertension can be divided into primary or 'essential' hypertension (for which no particular cause has been elucidated, although there is a familial tendency), and secondary hypertension.

Secondary hypertension may be caused by:

- Renal disease of whatever cause.
- Cushing's disease (*see* page 56).
- Conn's tumour, an adrenal adenoma secreting an excess of the mineralocorticosteroid, aldosterone.
- Phaeochromocytoma, a tumour of the adrenal medulla secreting excess catecholamines.
- Acromegaly, a tumour of the pituitary secreting excess growth hormone.
- Coarctation of the aorta (*see* page 13).
- Pregnancy-associated hypertension, usually developing in the last trimester (pre-eclampsia or eclampsia).
- Drugs, for example the oral contraceptive pill and following clonidine withdrawal.
- Following the ingestion of tyramine-containing foods (e.g. cheese) in those patients on monoamine oxidase inhibitors for depression.

Hypertension may also be divided into mild, moderate or severe, according to the levels of the blood pressure. The most severe, now known as accelerated hypertension, was formerly termed malignant hypertension as this described the previously poor prognosis of the condition, which, if untreated, lead to the majority of patients dying within 6–12 months. The characteristic features are diastolic blood pressure greater than 140 mmHg, proteinuria and papilloedema of the optic disc on fundoscopy.

Hypertension may be further divided into labile and fixed blood pressure. All blood pressure may rise as a result of stress and then return to normal. Fixed elevation of the blood pressure (hypertension) may also be labile, but it fails to fall to 'normal' levels when the stress has passed. Recordings of the blood pressure over a 24 hour period have highlighted the variability of the blood pressure and the normal fall of blood pressure during sleep.

It is therefore not surprising that the blood pressure may rise in a patient apprehensive of dental treatment. For the most part, these fluctuations are of no importance. It must be remembered that hypertension *per se,* unless markedly elevated, is to a large extent asymptomatic, apart from its complications. Symptoms of anxiety and headaches are not those of hypertension.

Medical management

The aim is to decrease the risks associated with hypertension. Numerous trials have confirmed that this can, to a large extent, be achieved. However, there has been some disappointment that the decrease in heart disease has not been as dramatic as the effects of the treatment on the other complications of hypertension.

Initial treatment is directed at correction of obesity, reduction in salt and alcohol intake, as well as attention to other risk factors of cardiovascular disease, for example, cholesterol. In addition, a variety of different therapies may be employed.

In general five groups of drugs are used:

- Diuretics.
- Beta-blockers.
- Calcium antagonists (calcium channel blockers).
- Vasodilators.
- Angiotensin converting enzyme inhibitors (ACEI).

The dental practitioner should be aware of the more common or more serious side effects of antihypertensive therapy:

- Postural hypotension – this may occur with a number of antihypertensive drugs.
- Bradycardia, in association with beta-blockers, with the consequent result that the tachycardia, in response to stress or shock, may not be seen.
- Flushing, which occurs with some calcium antagonists.

- Angioedema, a rare but serious complication with ACEI.
- Bronchospasm, in patients on beta-blockers who have a history of asthma or chronic obstructive airway diseases.

Anaphylaxis

Although anaphylaxis is not a cardiovascular disorder it is associated with cardiovascular signs and symptoms and is included in this section for completeness. Anaphylaxis is the symptom complex accompanying the acute reaction to a foreign substance to which a person has previously been sensitised. The term anaphylactoid reaction is used to describe reactions clinically identical to anaphylaxis but in which the mechanism is non-immunological or unknown.

Sensitisation occurs following exposure to an allergenic substance, subsequent contact or re-exposure to that substance results in an antigen/antibody reaction and the release of histamine and other mediators.

The period between the exposure and the development of symptoms is variable. It may be immediate, occurring within 30 minutes, or delayed, and the reaction may be mild, severe or fatal.

An immediate allergic response, if severe, may result in what is termed 'anaphylactic shock'. The most common causes are vaccines, insect stings, certain drugs such as antibiotics, iron injections, anti-inflammatory analgesics – especially aspirin containing compounds, and heparin and occurs in people who have been previously sensitised when challenged with the sensitising agent again.

Anaphylactic shock is an acute systemic reaction. There is marked apprehension and a 'feeling of impending doom', there may be a generalised urticaria or oedema, and back pain. There is vascular collapse with a drop in the blood pressure (hypotension), an increased heart rate (tachycardia), severe bronchospasm and generalised increased tissue permeability (angio-edema). The loss of plasma into the tissues, thereby reducing the effective blood volume, is the major cause of shock. In some cases there is oedema of the mouth, larynx, and laryngeal stridor with severe difficulty in breathing.

These symptoms may develop in a matter of 1–2 minutes.

Treatment

Prompt management is imperative. The airway must be maintained and supplementary oxygen given. Emergency treatment includes laying the patient flat with the head in a lateral position and raising the feet. This position will help to maintain the airway and aid the restoration of the blood pressure. If respiration has ceased an endotracheal tube should be inserted and the patient ventilated.

Adrenaline should be given intramuscularly 0.5–1mg (0.5–1ml adrenaline injection 1/1,000) and repeated every 10 minutes, according to the response of pulse and blood pressure, until improvement occurs.

The patient should be admitted to hospital for further treatment and assessment.

2 Disorders of the Blood

Haemophilia

The term 'haemophilia' was given to the disorder by Johann Schonlein in 1820, although the condition had been known from early times and recognised because of the Jewish practice of circumcision. The first description appeared in the Salem Gazette regarding a young man, Isaac Zoll, who died at the age of 25 years as a result of exsanguination, as had his five brothers before him. His father had two wives and several children with each, those who had died were all children with his first wife.

Haemophilia affects all races and is inherited as an X-linked recessive factor (14). Because it is transmitted on the X-chrosome it affects only males, females, having two X-chrosomes, are protected. The incidence in males is 1:10,000. It can very rarely affect a female if she is the offspring of an affected father and a mother who carries the trait. All daughters of haemophiliacs are carriers and their sons will have a 50% chance of either being normal or haemophiliac and their daughters will have a 50% chance of either being normal or a carrier. In about 80% of males there is a positive family history.

Fertility in affected males is reduced, therefore one would expect a decline in the number of people affected. However, there seems to be a relatively high mutation rate, as a significant number of patients have no affected relative.

In 1936, Patek and Taylor extracted a substance from platelet-free plasma of normal individuals which when given to a haemophiliac promoted clotting. This was found to be a globulin and it was a deficiency of this globulin (AHG) that prevented clotting in the haemophiliac. The factor involved was termed factor VIII and the condition called haemophilia A.

The process of clotting of the blood is a complex mechanism which begins with the conversion of fibrinogen to fibrin by the action of thrombin. Prothrombin may be converted into thrombin either by a series of reactions involving factors VIII and IX or by tissue damage and the action of factor VII. Thus results the cascade mechanism of blood coagulation.

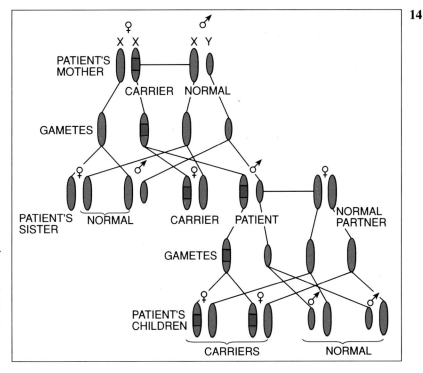

14 X-linked recessive pattern of inheritance. The abnormal gene is situated on the X-chromosome, the defect therefore is in the male but not the female, except in the rare event of her being homozygous (drawn by S. Davenport).

Haemophilia A

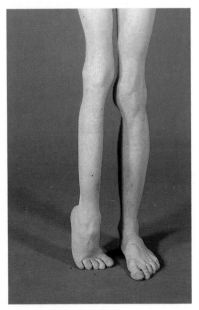

Haemophilia A is an X-linked disorder caused by deficiency of factor VIII (**14**). Bleeding may occur from the umbilical cord within the first few days of life. In severe forms there may be death in infancy from intracranial bleeding.

The degree of severity varies, but tends to be constant in a given family, and depends on the level of factor VIII in the plasma; it appears to run in a cyclical pattern, with periods of little or no bleeding. Those with over 25% of normal factor VIII activity may lead normal lives except for major trauma. Those with 6–25% are only mildly affected, while those with 1–5% are moderately to severely affected by minor trauma and experience spontaneous bleeding into the joints (haemarthrosis) (**15**). Those with less than 1% have multiple haemarthroses and may be severely handicapped as a result of damage to the joints. In children, there may also be damage to the growth centres at the ends of the long bones.

15 Chronic joint changes in a haemophiliac man due to recurrent haemarthroses which has resulted in grossly deformed knees, pes cavus (contraction of the foot) and shortening of the leg (courtesy of Dr J. Leslie).

Medical management

Prevention of trauma whenever possible is important, particularly when the child starts to become active. Replacement therapy must be carried out when bleeding occurs in order to prevent pain and permanent disabilities as a result of degenerative changes in the joints, muscle atrophy and osteoporosis. Factor VIII concentrates are now available and treatment in the home is therefore possible thus avoiding time off school and work. This has changed the lives of the younger generation of haemophiliacs and it is hoped that fewer deformities will occur. It is, however, still important that these patients are regularly monitored at their haemophiliac centre.

Although there has been a considerable improvement in the quality of life for those with haemophilia, it has been found that a large number of patients who received concentrated blood factors in certain regions before 1985 are now affected with the human immunodeficiency virus (HIV) causing acquired immune deficiency syndrome (AIDS). Since then all blood products in the UK have been screened and the risk of further patients becoming infected is very small. Hepatitis B carrier status is also more common in people with haemophilia, because until recently these viruses could not be inactivated by pasteurisation without destroying the coagulation factors, so contaminated factor VIII was administered.

An added complication is the development of inhibitors which inactivate factor VIII. The action of these inhibitors is to neutralise any factor VIII which is administered. Treatment can therefore only be given if the condition is life-threatening, when excessively large amounts of factor VIII are necessary.

It is important that the education of children with haemophilia is not neglected, as most types of manual work are contraindicated.

Dental care

In view of the large number of haemophiliac patients who are now affected with HIV and hepatitis virus, it is essential that appropriate precautions are taken to prevent cross-infection:

- Preventive treatment is extremely important, along with regular dental reviews.
- Supplementary fluorides should be prescribed if water fluoridation is inadequate.
- Topical fluorides should be applied at regular intervals.
- Bite-wing radiographs should be taken at regular intervals in order to detect caries at an early stage.
- Pulp treatment of primary molars, if indicated, is required in order to avoid extractions.
- Primary teeth when shed in the normal way cause little or no haemorrhage. However, if very mobile, extraction may be necessary because constant movement may cause trauma of the soft tissues and bleeding.

- Local anaesthetic infiltrations or intraligamentous injections are unlikely to cause problems. Never give inferior dental nerve blocks as bleeding in the pterygomandibular region may result in asphyxia.
- Extractions require admission to hospital and there must be adequate replacement therapy and careful monitoring of factor VIII levels. Routine therapy with the anti-fibrinolytic agents, tranexamic acid, or epsilon aminocaproic acid prior to and for a few days following the procedure will significantly reduce the requirement for replacement of factor VIII.
- Medications containing aspirin (salicylates) must not be prescribed as they may cause gastric bleeding. Paracetamol compounds may be used safely. Non-steroidal anti-inflammatory drugs (NSAIDs) are also contraindicated.
- Patients should carry a haemophiliac card which records details such as factor deficiency and level, the presence or absence of inhibitors and the telephone number of their haemophilia centre.

Christmas disease (haemophilia B)

In 1947 it was found that not all patients thought to be haemophiliacs responded to the addition of anti-haemophiliac globulin (AHG). A number of different workers in 1952 found that there was another factor termed factor IX. The condition was called haemophilia B and is now known as Christmas disease after the name of the first patient proved to have the condition. Female carriers of this condition also have a tendency to bleed. Inhibitors of factor IX may complicate management.

Medical management

Replacement therapy with fresh frozen plasma or freeze dried factor IX concentrate is necessary if there has been any trauma or bleeding.

Dental care

Similar precautions as with haemophilia A, but using factor IX instead.

Von Willebrand's Disease (Vascular Haemophilia)

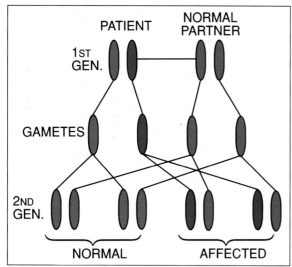

16 Autosomal dominant pattern of inheritance. Half the children of the affected parent exhibit the disease (drawn by S. Davenport).

In 1931 a further condition was described in which there was abnormal bleeding. Von Willebrand's disease is probably the second most common form of hereditary clotting disorder. The condition affects both males and females and is inherited as a dominant trait (**16**). Those affected have large tortuous capillaries, a low level of factor VIII and the condition may simulate haemophilia. These patients also have defective platelets which do not adhere to each other.

Bleeding from the gingiva, the mucosa of the nose and the gastro-intestinal tract is common and there is prolonged bleeding following trauma or surgery.

Medical management

If bleeding occurs fresh plasma may be effective, but the results are variable and it may be necessary to give cryoprecipitate. Bleeding can often be controlled by the use of the fibrinolytic inhibitor, tranexamic acid.

Dental care

Preventive treatment, whenever possible, will reduce admission to hospital for extractions.

Thrombocytopenia

Thrombocytopenia is caused by a reduction in the number of platelets (normal range $150-400 \times 10^9$/litre) in the bloodstream and results in petechial haemorrhages (purpura) into the skin, mucous membranes (**17, 18**) and viscera, with haematemesis (blood in the vomit), haematuria (blood in the urine) and malaena (blood in stools).

Platelets are formed in the bone marrow from megakaryocytes, they are released into the bloodstream and survive for about 7–10 days. The reduction in the number in thrombocytopenia may be due to failure of production, increased rate of destruction or increased utilisation.

Acute immune thrombocytopenic purpura occurs in children and is often preceded by an upper respiratory tract infection. Usually, recovery occurs within a few weeks and treatment is not necessary, although some patients may require a short course of steroids.

Intravenous immunoglobulin therapy may reverse the condition, but a splenectomy may be necessary.

Other causes include either a reduction in platelet production caused by leukaemic infiltration into the bone marrow, drugs, and infection. There may be a decrease in the survival of the platelets as a result of certain drugs (quinine, heparin and digoxin) and occasionally following massive blood transfusions.

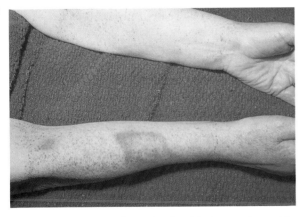

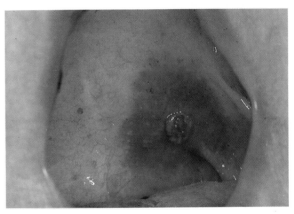

17 Petechial haemorrhages in the skin in a patient with thrombocytopenia. The right arm appears to be more severely affected, but this is a result of placing a cuff to take the blood pressure.

18 Sub-mucosal haemorrhage in the palate of a patient with thrombocytopenia.

Dental care

The platelet count should be estimated prior to extractions or other surgical procedures. If the platelet count is low the patient should be referred to their physician as the administration of platelet concentrates may be necessary to cover the period of surgery.

Provided the platelet count is above 50×10^9 / litre prolonged post-extraction haemorrhage is unlikely.

Anaemia

Anaemia is defined as a reduction of the red cell volume or haemoglobin concentration below the range of values occurring in healthy individuals. Anaemia is not a specific entity but an indication or manifestation of underlying disease and it is essential to ascertain the cause.

The main clinical features of anaemia are:

- Pallor which is best detected in the conjunctiva, nail bed or in the mucous membrane of the mouth. Pallor of the skin is deceptive as this can occur in fair-skinned people and is difficult to detect in coloured races.
- Tiredness, listlessness and fatigue.
- Breathlessness which occurs as a result of tissue hypoxia. (In severe anaemia, congestive cardiac failure may occur.)
- Angina pectoris may occur in older age groups.

Anaemias are described by the morphological characteristics of the red cells, as follows:

- Acute post-haemorrhagic anaemia (normocytic and normochromic). Blood loss may be caused by trauma; peptic ulcer and other gastro-intestinal ulceration; or haemorrhagic disease.
- Iron deficiency anaemia (microcytic and hypochromic). This may result from: chronic blood loss as a result of gastrointestinal bleeding or excessive loss of blood at menstruation; defective iron absorption; or dietary deficiency. Malabsorption may occur in infants as milk contains little iron. This may also occur in the elderly due to inadequate iron in the diet.

Following iron therapy, all signs and symptoms disappear.

- Megaloblastic anaemia (macrocytic). This is due to a deficiency of folic acid, Vitamin B_{12}, or both. Its causes include malabsorption, pernicious anaemia, gastric disease, or intestinal malabsorption.
- Haemolytic anaemia (normochromic and normocytic). Red cells normally spend 100–120 days in the circulation, however, there may be an increase in the rate of destruction of red cells due to intrinsic defects in the red cells or extra-corpuscular factors acting on normal cells.
- Haemolytic anaemias due to haemoglobinopathies.
- Anaemia due to chronic diseases; for example, chronic renal failure, rheumatoid arthritis.

Sickle cell anaemia

Sickle cell anaemia (HbSS) is an inherited autosomal recessive disorder that affects the red blood cells and occurs as a result of both parents carrying the gene (**19**). The condition occurs predominantly in people of African, Afro-Caribbean, Asian and Mediterranean origin. The name sickle cell is derived from the fact that the red blood cells take on the form of a sickle shape instead of the normal spherical form. The disease was described by Dr Herrick, an American, in 1910, however, prior to this the disease had been given different tribal names in Africa.

In sickle cell anaemia the red blood cells containing sickle haemoglobin, haemoglobin S, have a life of only about 30–60 days. As a result of their deformity, the red cells may be unable to flow normally on certain occasions. They become clumped together, blocking

19

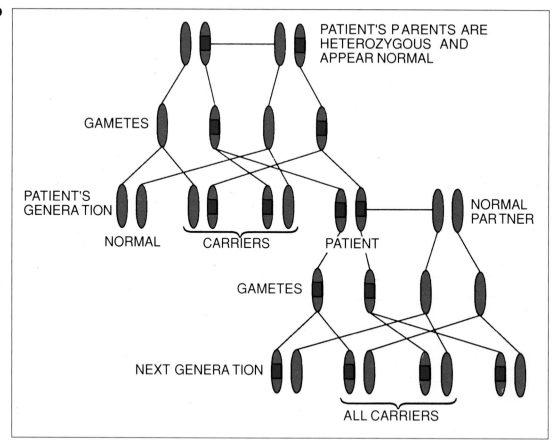

19 Autosomal recessive inheritance in which the patient inherits the abnormal gene from both parents who are heterozygous and carriers. All the patient's children will be carriers (drawn by S. Davenport).

small blood vessels, which leads to pain and, if there is prolonged reduction in the blood supply, necrosis of the tissue supplied may result.

This is a severe chronic haemolytic anaemia which varies in its severity from person to person. Symptoms do not usually occur until the end of the first year of life and include:

- Tiredness, weakness, breathlessness on exertion and pallor.
- Painful joints and painful swelling of the hands and feet due to the occlusion of small blood vessels (hand–foot syndrome).
- Lowered resistance to infection. Chronic leg ulcers are common in adolescent and early adult life. There is also an increased incidence of pneumococcal meningitis and septicaemia.
- Growth retardation and failure to thrive.
- An enlarged spleen, which has reduced function in early childhood. Later, as a result of repeated infarctions, it becomes small and fibrotic.
- Impairment of renal function by progressive ischaemia.
- Possible retinal and conjunctival damage.

Acute symptoms may occur as a result of sudden sickling and are termed 'crises'. The frequency depends on the severity of the disease and predisposing factors, the most common being stress, infection, anoxia and emotional upsets. There is excruciating pain and the person may be in a state of shock.

Medical management

None is necessary except during crises. However, the avoidance of cold, infection and dehydration is advised. Iron therapy is not indicated. Dehydration and acidosis must be actively corrected intravenously. Codeine is often sufficient for the control of the pain and discomfort. Hospital admission is usually necessary during a crisis so that antibiotics and fluid balance may be maintained.

Dental care

All black patients should be tested routinely for sickle cell disease prior to a general anaesthetic so that precautions may be taken in order to avoid a crisis as a result of inadequate oxygenation. The level of haemoglobin A should also be investigated before extractions or surgery and haemoglobin S should be less than 30%. Local anaesthesia should be used in preference to general anaesthesia whenever possible. Antibiotics should be given to avoid or control infection.

Sickle cell trait

The heterozygous form or sickle cell trait (HbAS) is usually symptomless and the person may be unaware of the condition. About 8% of American black people have the trait and there is a high incidence among African people. About 1% of people living in Britain are carriers.

Thalassaemia

Thalassaemia is one of the most important inherited disorders of haemoglobin synthesis. The name thalassaemia derives from the Greek word 'thalassa' meaning sea, i.e. the Mediterranean. It occurs in many parts of the world, but particularly in the Mediterranean countries such as Cyprus, Turkey, Italy and Greece, and in the Middle and Far East. There are about 700 affected people in Cyprus, 12,000 in Italy and 3,000 in Greece. The disease is sometimes called Mediterranean anaemia or Cooley's anaemia. Like the sickle cell gene, that of thalassaemia appears to be associated with an increased resistance to malaria. This may account for the geographic distribution and its persistence.

The condition may be heterozygous (thalassaemia minor or B-thalassaemia trait) or homozygous (thalassaemia major). Those with the heterozygous form are healthy and are unaware of the condition. Half the offspring of a carrier and a normal person will be carriers. However, the offspring of two persons with the trait will be one affected, one normal and two carriers. Fetal blood sampling at 16–22 weeks gestation or trophoblastic biopsy as early as 9–12 weeks permits the diagnosis of thalassaemia major and termination may be offered.

Approximately 1 in 7 Cypriots are carriers, 1 in 10 South Italians, 1 in 20 Turks and Indians, 1 in 12 Greeks, and 1 in 1,000 British. The British carriers are mostly of Cypriot origin, the rest are Italian, Greek, Chinese, Pakistani and Indian.

The condition is usually apparent when the child is a few months old. The child becomes pale and weak and fails to thrive; this is due to the anaemia secondary to haemolysis.

Enlargement of the spleen (splenomegaly) is common and jaundice and leg ulcers have also been reported to occur.

There is a wide variety of radiographic bone abnormalities consisting of large medullary cavities, thin cortices and generalised osteoporosis due to the increased stimulus to produce haematopoietic tissue. In addition there is expansion of the medullary cavities of the facial bones, which become more pronounced with age and give rise to expansion of the maxilla, creating protrusion of the middle third of the face.

Medical management

The minor form may be misdiagnosed as an iron deficiency anaemia and treated with iron. In the major form, transfusions are necessary on a regular basis or the life expectancy will only be a few years.

As the red blood cells contain iron, with the destruction of the blood cells there is a gradual accumulation of iron in the body which may cause complications in the liver, pancreas and heart. The drug, desferrioxamine, which acts as an iron chelating agent, prevents this gradual accumulation of iron and if it is given by injection on a daily basis may help to prolong life.

Dental care

The gradual expansion of the maxilla obviously has repercussions as far as orthodontic management is concerned. General anaesthesia should also be avoided.

Leukaemia

Leukaemia is a malignant disease in which there is widespread proliferation of white blood cells and their precursors. It is, in essence, a cancer of the marrow resulting in an abnormality of the quality and quantity of cells that enter the circulation.

It is the most common form of childhood cancer and accounts for about a third of such cancers diagnosed in children each year. The age of onset is usually about 3–4 years. Although the cause of leukaemia is unknown, there appears to be a genetic disposition and certain chromosomal abnormalities have a higher incidence. Those with Down's syndrome have an increased risk of developing leukaemia. Radiation and certain chemicals are also implicated in a small percentage of cases.

The condition may be first apparent orally and the dentist must be alerted to spontaneous haemorrhage from the gingivae and petechiae (**20**).

The leukaemias are classified according to the rapidity of the disease and the type of cell involved. The diagnosis of the cell-type involved is essential as the treatment and prognosis of the various types differ:

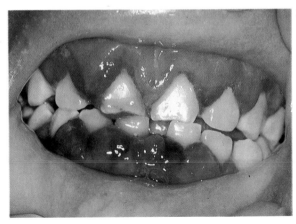

20 Oral appearance of a patient with acute myeloblastic leukaemia, showing infiltration of the gingivae and spontaneous haemorrhage.

- Chronic leukaemia:
  Chronic myelocytic (CML).
  Chronic lymphocytic (CLL)
- Acute leukaemia:
  Acute myeloblastic (AML).
  Acute lymphoblastic (ALL).
  Acute monoblastic (AMOL).

Chronic myelocytic leukaemia (CML)

This disease occurs in middle-age most often in those exposed to radiation. There is no cure for this condition although chemotherapy may slow its progress. There is progressive anaemia and thrombocytopenia and death occurs usually within 3–5 years.

Chronic lymphocytic leukaemia (CLL)

This disease occurs in later life. Most of the cells in the bloodstream are mature lymphocytes and result in anaemia and thrombocytopenia. Death usually occurs because of anaemia and infection in 3–5 years.

Acute leukaemia

The three types (listed above) closely resemble each other. Primitive white cells replace the mature ones and the polymorph count is reduced (agranulocytosis). These immature cells are incompetent and this results in the body being unable to cope with infection.

The onset is usually sudden with a high fever, generalised bleeding tendency and infective lesions of the mouth and throat. Indeed, the patient may seek dental treatment as a result of infection and gingivitis.

Medical management

The aim of treatment is to remove the abnormal cells from the blood and the bone marrow in order to achieve a remission. This can be achieved in about 90% of patients by the use of chemotherapy. In early series it was found that there was a relapse in around half the children treated who had had a haematological remission. This relapse was due to leukaemic cells infiltrating the central nervous system. The remission rate was improved dramatically by irradiation of the central nervous system and intrathecal methotrexate. Maintenance treatment is necessary for about 2–3 years. The prognosis for boys is worse than that for girls because of testicular disease. Bone marrow transplantation may be contemplated when the patient is in remission.

Dental care

No treatment should be carried out until the patient is in remission unless there is an emergency and then this should be treated conservatively by the use of antibiotics and analgesics. Multiple painful ulcers may occur and these are liable to become secondarily infected. Swabbing the mouth with an antibacterial solution such as chlorhexidine and antifungal therapy may help to prevent this. Many patients have acute nausea when a high dosage of drugs is being used to induce remission and oral hygiene procedures are difficult. Mouthwashes with local anaesthetic properties used before mealtimes may be beneficial.

Once in remission, dental treatment may be carried out, but inferior dental blocks are contraindicated as there is the possibility of deep haemorrhage. The bleeding time and platelet count should be checked before extractions or extensive scaling.

Leukaemic patients are susceptible to all infections, and are often maintained on prophylactic antibiotics; if viral infections, such as herpetic gingivo-stomatitis, develop then intravenous or oral acyclovir is required. Candidal infections may also occur and should be treated with amphotericin B, nystatin locally or, if severe or resistant, fluconazole.

3 Respiratory Disorders

Chronic Obstructive Pulmonary Disease (Chronic Bronchitis)

Chronic bronchitis used to be called the 'English disease'. In adults it is defined as a productive cough of 2–3 months duration occurring each year for two or more years. It usually develops as a result of prolonged infection or irritation of the lungs, by either chemical or physical means. Coal dust, fumes and air pollution may all contribute to the condition, but cigarette smoking is probably the commonest cause, and the effects of passive smoking should not be forgotten. With the introduction of smokeless zones, better housing and living conditions, and the use of antibiotics there has been a reduction in the incidence.

Although children may be diagnosed as having bronchitis, the cough is usually due to some underlying systemic condition or an early manifestation of asthma. Chronic chest infection is likely to develop in a child who gets bronchitis in the first year of life and never fully recovers.

The chief symptom is a cough which is usually worse at night and may result in a sore chest.

Children who have had severe whooping cough may later develop chronic respiratory disorders due to bronchiectasis. Immunisation in infancy may avoid such complications.

Medical management

Bed rest and antipyretics may be necessary until the fever subsides. The underlying cause of the cough should be treated and antibiotics administered where appropriate.

Dental care

General anaesthesia should be avoided in severe bronchitics, particularly in the winter months.

Bronchiectasis

Bronchiectasis is the dilatation of the bronchi. Rarely it occurs as a congenital condition, possibly due to arrested development. Usually it is acquired as a result of destruction of the bronchial walls due to infection if treatment is delayed or when there are resistant organisms, or if there has been inhalation of noxious chemicals. Cystic fibrosis is probably the most common cause in children (see page 39). Clinically, the condition varies according to the severity and in many cases it may be asymptomatic. In more severe cases there is a productive cough with purulent sputum. The condition follows a course of acute exacerbations and remissions.

Medical management

Control of the infection by appropriate antibiotics and postural drainage with physiotherapy.

Dental care

Patients may attend the dentist because of halitosis and should be referred for further investigation if no oral cause is found. General anaesthesia should be avoided unless absolutely essential.

Asthma

Asthma is probably the commonest cause of recurrent respiratory problems in children. It has been known from ancient times. There were descriptions in Egyptian medical records from around 3,000 BC. The word 'asthma' is derived from the Greek word for 'panting' or 'gasping'. Between 5 and 10% of schoolchildren have some evidence of asthma. Prior to puberty, asthma is twice as common in boys as in girls. After adolescence the incidence is about equal.

The symptoms, such as wheeze and breathlessness, result from bronchoconstriction. First, there is a tightening of the bronchial smooth muscles, followed by swelling (oedema) of the tissues lining the bronchi. Finally, there is an increase in the mucous secretions. This results in a decrease in the diameter of the airway and causes wheezing. There may also be a dry non-productive hacking cough which may be exhausting and dominate the picture. The initial attacks are usually precipitated by respiratory infections. In a severe attack the child will sit with the shoulders hunched forward, labouring hard to breathe, the accessory muscles of respiration are used, the chest moves with each respiratory effort, and the nostrils may flare. The noise of breathing is easily heard and the child may appear anxious. However, in very severe asthma, wheezing may not be heard because the respiration is so shallow, and this may be a trap for the unwary.

The aetiology is little understood; biological, immunological, infectious, endocrine and psychological factors have all been implicated. There also seems to be a genetic component, although this has not been proved.

Asthma can start at any age but occurs most commonly in children. If wheezing occurs before 1 year of age it may be due to a food allergy. Wheezing that starts between 1 and 5 years of age is most likely to be due to allergy to house dust mites (dermatophagoides — 'eater of skin'), pollens and moulds. After 5 years of age the cause is more likely to be due to pollens and grasses. In mild forms of the disease the child often gets better by the end of his or her school days. However, some children will get increasingly more severe forms of the disease. With effective therapy, the majority of children may have complete relief, or at least a reduction in the severity of their attacks. Unfortunately, some children may get permanent chest deformities (see **21**).

Medical management

Avoidance of known allergens is important. Some children require regular use of bronchodilators and inhaled steroids. Inhaled disodium chromoglycate may prevent attacks by preventing the release of histamine. It is particularly beneficial in asthma which has an allergic basis and in exercise-induced asthma. It is important that children participate in various sporting activities, but short periods of activity rather than endurance tests. Prophylactic therapy may be necessary before exercise in such children.

More severe forms require prompt treatment with nebulised bronchodilators to achieve penetration to the airways as well as intravenous steroids and/or aminophylline. The duration of an attack is not a guide to its severity and many of the deaths caused by asthma are due to failure of the patient, and occasionally the physician, to appreciate the severity of the attack. In severe attacks, besides the dyspnoea the patient may exhibit restlessness, exhaustion, a tachycardia (over 110/minute) and often 'pulsus paradoxus' (reduction in arterial and pulse pressure with inspiration).

Such patients should *not* be sedated as it may depress respiration. There is also a risk of pneumothorax in asthmatics. This diagnosis should be considered in any asthmatic whose breathing deteriorates.

Prednisolone may be given orally in short courses during acute exacerbations. In a few patients long-term maintenance may be necessary. The duration of oral steroids should be as short as possible in order to avoid the long-term sequelae of steroid therapy, especially growth retardation in children, diabetes, peptic ulceration, infection and possible mental changes.

Dental care

There are no problems with local anaesthetics. However, for severe asthmatics, if a general anaesthetic is required admission to hospital may be advisable. If the patient is on oral steroids and surgery is required, it is necessary to consult the patient's physician, as an increase in steroids may be necessary.

If a severe asthmatic attack occurs in the dental surgery *prompt* treatment is required. The patient should be seated upright in the chair and oxygen administered. Hydrocortisone (200mg) should be injected intravenously and a bronchodilator inhaler given.

Cystic Fibrosis

Cystic fibrosis is an inherited condition and was first noted by Fanconi in 1936. In 1938 Professor Anderson, a pathologist, reported a series of infants who all died of lung disease before their first birthday. She noticed that the pancreas was involved as well as the lungs. As there were cystic changes in the pancreas and fibrous scarring she named the disease cystic fibrosis of the pancreas. She also theorised that the disorder prevented the absorption of vitamin A. In 1945 Farber suggested the name 'mucoviscidosis' for the condition, as all the mucus-producing glands produced thick mucus that caused obstruction of the flow of secretions from the ducts.

Cystic fibrosis is an autosomal recessive disorder of the exocrine glands and occurs in approximately 1 in 2,000 births in Caucasians, much less frequently in Black children and extremely rarely in Oriental children. Males and females are equally affected. Males tend to live for longer and most are infertile. Recent research has localised the cystic fibrosis gene on the long arm of chromosome 7. About 4–5% of the population are carriers and there is a chance of 1 in 4 of offspring of two carriers being affected (*see* **19**).

About 10% of children with cystic fibrosis are born with obstruction of the ileum by meconium (meconium ileus) and a distended abdomen.

The lungs are invariably involved and there is a non-productive cough that leads to acute respiratory infection, bronchopneumonia, bronchiectasis and lung abscesses. Recurrent chest infection is attributed to the lack of resistance of the respiratory epithelium because of failure of absorption of vitamin A. Mucus in the lung is not removed effectively so the small bronchioles become occluded, causing collapse of the distal alveoli; this may result in a 'barrel-chest' deformity and

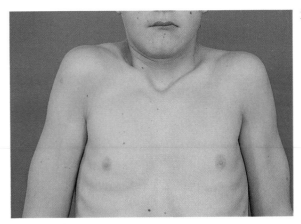

21

21 This boy has cystic fibrosis and exhibits a 'barrel-chest' deformity due to repeated respiratory infections. (Coincidentally he also has a deformity of his clavicles.)

development of the accessory muscles of respiration (**21**).

Involvement of the pancreas results in obstruction and the gland atrophies. Stools are frequent, bulky, greasy and have a foul odour because of the excretion of undigested fats. The patient may have a voracious appetite or fail to thrive as a result of chronic malabsorption syndrome due to pancreatic insufficiency. Diabetes may be an added complication as a result of progressive pancreatic damage. Cirrhosis of the liver may lead to defects of the clotting mechanism.

Confirmation of the diagnosis may be made by the family history, chronic pulmonary involvement and the absence of pancreatic enzymes; but specifically by determining the concentration of salt in sweat that has been chemically stimulated using the pilocarpine iontophoresis sweat test, as there is an elevation of chloride and sodium levels (sodium levels of more than 60 mmol/l). Although this test is diagnostic in children it is inaccurate in adults. In warm weather an active person may lose enough salt in the sweat to necessitate intravenous replacement.

Medical management

The disease pursues a relentless course and until recently the life expectancy was not much more than the second decade. However, with early diagnosis and treatment many patients may live well into the third and fourth decade.

Physiotherapy in the form of postural drainage is necessary three times a day to remove accumulated secretions and relieve bronchial obstruction. Antibiotic therapy is also necessary to prevent infection, and inhaled antibiotics may be especially beneficial. In the past, tetracycline was the antibiotic of choice. This should not be given to children under the age of 9 years, as the tetracycline is incorporated into the teeth, calcifying at that time, resulting in unsightly discolouration (**22, 23**).

There must also be modifications to the diet, administration of pancreatic enzymes and the addition of vitamins A, D, E and K. If patients are unable to maintain their weight it may be necessary to supplement feeding by a nasogastric tube or to start parenteral nutrition.

Heart and lung transplants have proved successful in a small group of patients with respiratory failure.

22

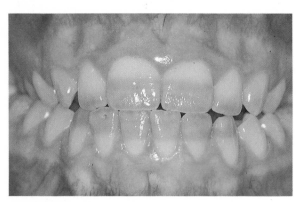

22 Discolouration of the permanent dentition in a girl with cystic fibrosis due to the administration of tetracycline until she was 1 year old, when the drug was changed.

23

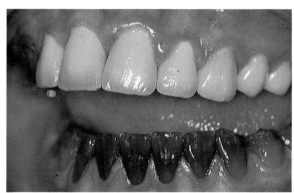

23 Older sister of the girl shown in **22**, who also had cystic fibrosis. Following eruption of her permanent teeth the link between tetracycline and the discolouration of her teeth was confirmed and tetracycline was discontinued in her 1-year-old sister. All her permanent upper teeth have been crowned and this was then followed by crowns in the lower arch.

Dental care

General anaesthesia should be avoided in view of the respiratory condition. Cirrhosis of the liver may result in a defect in the clotting mechanism and consequent bleeding following extractions or surgery.

4 Renal Disorders

Nephrotic Syndrome

Normally only a trace of protein escapes into the glomerular filtrate and most of it is re-absorbed in the proximal convoluted tubules, thus less than 200mg of protein appears in the urine over a period of 24 hours. Damage to the glomeruli may be manifested by a decrease in renal function, by chronic renal failure, or with significant proteinuria or both. When proteinuria exceeds 3g/24 hours, the term 'nephrotic syndrome' is applied. Associated with the loss of protein there is a concomitant fall in the serum albumin, dependent oedema (due to loss of osmotic pressure in the blood vessels) and hypercholesterolaemia.

There are a variety of causes, from primary renal disease with immune-complex mediated glomerulonephritis, to systemic disease, such as diabetes or amyloid. In children, the nephrotic syndrome is more common in boys than in girls in a ratio of 2:1, with the onset at 2–6 years of age, and is secondary to glomerulonephritis. The presenting symptom is usually oedema, particularly of the face and eyelids (**24**), and the lower extremities, the legs and the ankles. There is also an increased susceptibility to infection.

Nephrotic syndrome is, as its name implies, a syndrome, and it is important to ascertain the aetiology. A full drug history is essential as drugs may be incriminated in some patients. A renal biopsy may also be necessary.

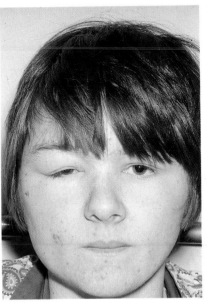

24

24 Young boy with oedema of the face and eyelids who has nephrotic syndrome.

Medical management

This may be divided into general and specific. General management is aimed at reduction of salt intake, diuretics and, if the serum albumin is very low, infusion of albumin is undertaken. In children with glomerulonephritis, steroids may be given. Resolution of the nephrotic state may be achieved (**25**), but relapses are not uncommon and further courses of steroids and other immunosuppressive therapy may be required. The condition usually resolves itself spontaneously towards the end of the second decade, although a few patients may progress to chronic renal failure.

In adults, immunosuppressive therapy may also be

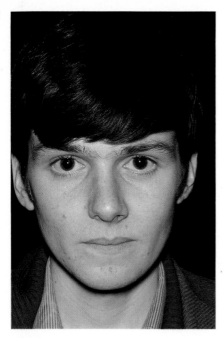

given to reverse the nephrosis if it is secondary to glomerulonephritis, while full supportive care is given to those with diabetic nephropathy, there being no specific therapy at that stage which will reverse the process.

Dental care

There is an increased susceptibility to infection. Pulp treatments in primary molar teeth are contraindicated and prophylactic antibiotic cover is advisable before extractions. There should be consultation with the patient's physician if the patient is on steroids, as these may need to be increased, particularly if a general anaesthetic is necessary.

25 The boy shown in **24** following treatment.

Chronic Renal Failure

Chronic renal failure may be due to renal hypoplasia, reflux nephropathy, hereditary nephritis, polycystic kidneys, outflow obstruction, chronic glomerulonephritis, diabetes or long-standing hypertension.

As the disease progresses there is a gradual loss of nephrons, which results in a loss of renal function. Large amounts of dilute urine may be passed and such patients must have an increased fluid intake to prevent dehydration. As a result of the loss of the glomerular filtration there is a build up of nitrogenous waste products. There may be nausea, anorexia and fatigue and the patients are extremely susceptible to infection and there is a risk of gastrointestinal haemorrhage. The patient is also susceptible to heart failure and pulmonary oedema. Oral ulceration and candidiasis may occur.

Medical management

Initially, dietary treatment is undertaken with restriction of salt, protein and potassium, depending on the degree of renal failure. Ultimately, dialysis may be necessary. Anaemia may be treated with erythropoietin.

Dental care

If a general anaesthetic cannot be avoided the patient should be hospitalised and intravenous fluids administered pre-operatively to prevent dehydration and salt depletion. There may also be abnormalities of the clotting mechanism. There is a risk that the mandible may fracture during extractions as a result of renal bone disease (renal osteodystrophy). Fortunately, with modern management of patients with chronic renal failure, this is now rare because of appropriate treatment with 'activated' vitamin D (1-alpha-hydroxycholecalciferol).

Dialysis

Two methods of dialysis are employed for patients with end-stage renal failure, either chronic intermittent haemodialysis or continuous ambulatory peritoneal dialysis.

Chronic intermittent haemodialysis is usually necessary every 2–3 days and generally takes about 3–5 hours for each session. An arteriovenous fistula is created, usually at the wrist, to provide increased superficial flow, thereby enabling the patient to be connected to the dialysis machine. Blood is withdrawn from the patient through the dialyser, where it is filtered and returned to the patient via another cannula. Heparin is administered during dialysis in order to prevent clotting in the extracorporeal circulation (**26**).

Continuous ambulatory peritoneal dialysis involves the exchange of metabolites, salt and water using the patient's own peritoneal membrane as a filter. A soft dialysis catheter is inserted into the peritoneal cavity, usually under local anaesthesia, 1.5–2.0 litres of fluid are run into the peritoneal cavity and left *in situ* for several hours and then run out and replaced with fresh fluid. This process is usually necessary 3–4 times a day, 7 days a week. The advantages of this method are that the patient can manage this form of therapy at home or at work and is independent of a hospital, diet is less restrictive and there is a more variable fluid allowance. However, there is a greater risk of infection due to access to the peritoneal cavity, and peritonitis may develop.

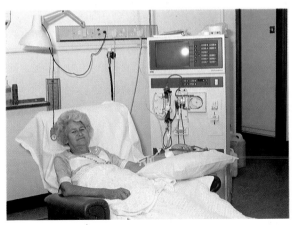

26 Patient undergoing dialysis.

Dental care

Patients on dialysis have a reduced immune response and are at particular risk from *Staphylococcus aureus*. In general, the administration of pre-operative antibiotics effective against staphylococci should be considered prior to invasive dental treatment.

As a result of the administration of heparin to prevent clotting during haemodialysis, there may be complications with extractions and oral surgery (*see* above). It has therefore been suggested that dental treatment should be carried out the day after dialysis when anticoagulation is minimal and benefits of dialysis are maximal. (The half life of heparin is 4 hours.) Some patients, however, are on long-term anticoagulation treatment with warfarin. The clotting time should always be checked prior to any surgery. Anaemia may also present a problem.

Bacteraemia can present risks if there is an arteriovenous shunt. General anaesthesia may also be hazardous to the patient because of associated hypertension, arteriosclerosis and anaemia.

Transplantation

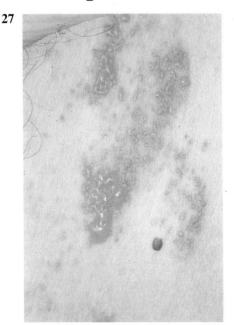

27 Herpes zoster infection in a patient who has received a kidney transplant and is on immunosuppressive drugs.

The most commonly transplanted organ today is the kidney; the long-term results are proving extremely successful and it is regarded as the optimum form of therapy. The quality of life is greatly improved and the patient is able to live a more normal existence when no longer requiring dialysis. A problem, as with any transplant (with the exception of transplantation between identical twins), is that of rejection since the donor organ is recognised as 'foreign' by the recipient. Antirejection therapy is required, initially in high doses and subsequently decreasing.

A wide variety of drugs have been used to suppress rejection including steroids, azathioprine, cyclosporin A and antilymphocytic globulin. As a consequence, the patient is more susceptible to infection and there is poor wound healing. Infection with herpes zoster is particularly common in those who are immunosuppressed (**27**).

If there is any degree of renal dysfunction, drugs which are excreted by the kidneys should be avoided. Chlorpropamide, metformin, nalidixic acid, nitrofurantoin, and tetracycline are all contraindicated.

Dental care

Patients who are awaiting renal transplants should be made dentally fit and any teeth with a doubtful prognosis removed. Antibiotics should be given to prevent transient bacteraemia and to avoid postoperative infection following surgical procedures. If the patient is on steroids, the physician should be consulted before a surgical procedure or a general anaesthetic is administered, as additional steroids will be necessary to prevent adrenal insufficiency.

Nystatin mouthwashes should be prescribed the day before a transplant operation and also post-operatively in order to avoid candidiasis which occurs in the immunosuppressed patient.

Gingival hyperplasia may occur in patients on cyclosporin A and nifedipine (**28**), which is similar to that in patients on phenytoin. Treatment is by removal of calculus and meticulous oral hygiene and, if necessary, a gingivectomy.

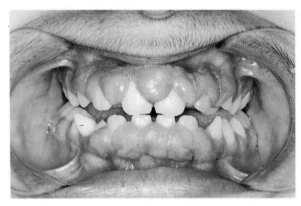

28 Gross gingival hyperplasia in a post kidney transplant patient who has significant hypertension and is on cyclosporin and nifedipine. In spite of good compliance with oral hygiene care, surgical reduction will probably be necessary.

5 Neoplasms and Neoplasm-like Lesions

Haemangiomas

Haemangiomas are developmental abnormalities or hamartomas. A hamartoma is a tumour-like malformation in which the tissues of a particular part are arranged haphazardly. The term was coined by Albrect in 1904 and comes from the Greek word 'hamartein' meaning 'to err'.

Various types of vascular anomalies are seen on the skin:

- The capillary haemangioma or spider naevus is small and aptly named. Its blood supply is usually from a single arteriole and it causes few problems. There may be an increase in their number during pregnancy or in association with alcoholic liver disease.

- The naevus flammeus, or port wine stain, has dilated capillaries and is flat and erythematous (**29**).
- Cavernous haemangiomas are less well circumscribed, non-encapsulated and tend to extend more deeply into the subcutaneous tissues and even into the underlying bone.

Haemangiomas grow with the child but then usually regress in size. Even with regression surgical treatment may be necessary. They may be of little significance apart from the aesthetic consideration, however, bone involvement should be suspected if there is early eruption of the teeth in the affected area, which could be due to an increased blood supply (**30**).

29

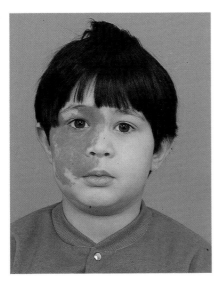

29 Haemangioma (port wine stain) affecting the right maxillary region.

30

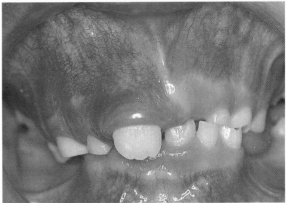

30 Intra-oral view of the boy in **29**. The right maxillary region appears redder and there is early eruption of the upper right central incisor which suggests an increased blood supply in that area.

Medical management

If the haemangioma affects the face it may be masked by cosmetics. Surgery may be necessary to improve the appearance. More recently, the use of lasers for superficial lesions has resulted in quite marked improvement.

Dental care

Preventive treatment is of the utmost importance, as extraction of a tooth in an involved area may cause uncontrollable haemorrhage. Radiographs may not reveal the presence of bone involvement.

All preventive measures should be taken (*see* Chapter 15), including bite-wing radiographs at regular intervals in order to detect early carious lesions. If caries has resulted in pulpal exposure in the primary dentition the teeth should be pulp-treated. Endodontic treatment may be necessary in the permanent dentition to avoid extractions. If extractions are unavoidable the patient should be hospitalised and cross-matched blood available.

Sturge–Weber Syndrome (Encephalotrigeminal Angiomatosis)

Sturge–Weber syndrome is of unknown aetiology. The lesion, which is usually unilateral, is a congenital haemangioma (port wine stain) affecting the trigeminal area of the skin of the face and neck and the mucous membrane (**31,32**). The condition, however, also involves the meninges and the choroid, resulting in convulsions, intellectual impairment and even hemiparesis. There may be minimal mental impairment, but this is likely to be progressive and in many cases it may not be possible to achieve independent living.

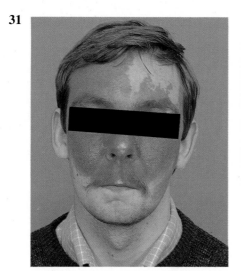

31 Capillary haemangioma involving both maxillae and the right frontal region in this young man with Sturge–Weber syndrome.

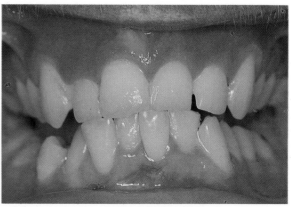

32 Intra-oral view of the man in **31** showing increased vascularity in the maxillary region.

Medical management

Anticonvulsant drugs may be necessary to control epileptic fits. The appearance may be improved by cosmetics or laser treatment.

Dental care

Preventive treatment is of the utmost importance as extractions in an area affected by the haemangioma may result in uncontrollable bleeding. Evidence of involvement of the bone may not be detectable on radiographs.

Histiocytosis X

Although an uncommon group of diseases, histiocytosis X is an important disease entity to the dentist because of its predilection for the orofacial structures. It is characterised by the infiltration of histiocytes and eosinophils into various tissues and was subdivided into three groups: a localised form, known as eosinophilic granuloma; a chronic disseminated type, known as Hand–Schuller–Christian disease; and an acute form, referred to as Letterer–Siwe disease with multiple soft tissue involvement.

Although there are various clinical manifestations of the condition the histopathological appearance is similar, and Lichenstein in 1953 suggested the single term histiocytosis X be used.

The localised form is the mildest form of the disease and may occur at any age, with a peak incidence in children and young adults. Although any bone may be affected, the skull and the mandible are common sites (**33,34**). It appears as a well-defined radiolucent lesion in the bone but may only become apparent as a result of invasion of the soft tissues.

The chronic disseminated form of the disease usually affects children over the age of 3 years. The classic triad of exophthalmos, diabetes insipidus and multiple bone lesions are seldom found in the same child.

The acute disseminated form may affect almost any tissue in the body, occurs in children less than 3 years of age, and may be present at birth. Clinically, there are cutaneous lesions resembling seborrhoeic eczema (**35**), hepatosplenomegaly, otitis externa or media, anaemia, haemorrhage, lymphadenopathy and osteolytic bone lesions.

33

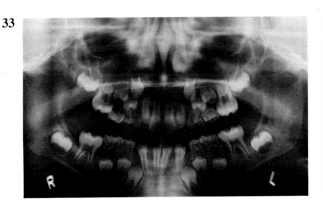

34

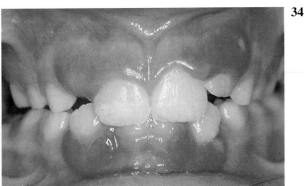

33 Orthopantomogram of child with histiocytosis X. There are extensive areas of rarefaction and bone loss mesial to the upper permanent first molars and in the lower incisor region.

34 Intra-oral view of patient in **33**. There is considerable inflammation in the upper lateral and lower incisor regions which is unexplained by the low level of plaque.

35

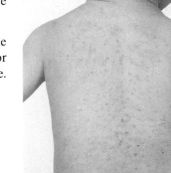

35 A 10-month-old baby with cutaneous lesions of histiocytosis X that resemble seborrhoeic eczema. This is the acute disseminated form and proved fatal in this child.

Medical management

The condition is no longer regarded as malignant, so there is a less aggressive approach to management than in the past.

Localised lesions may resolve and should be kept under observation. Intralesional corticosteroid injections several times over a few weeks may be beneficial.

Where there are multiple lesions oral steroids may also be effective, but this may result in failure of growth and immunosuppression. The prognosis for this form, despite treatment, is still poor.

Dental care

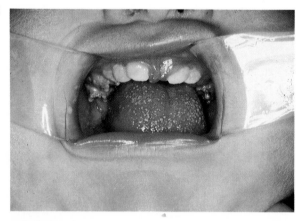

36

Histiocytosis X should be suspected if there is pain, gingivitis and tooth mobility (**36**), and radiolucent areas in the bone. The patient should be referred for investigation of lesions elsewhere in the body.

36 Intra-oral view of the baby in **35**, who has premature eruption of his primary canine and molar teeth, which are abnormally formed, very mobile and 'floating' in the soft tissue.

Hodgkin's Disease

This condition was first described by Dr Thomas Hodgkin in 1832. Its aetiology is unknown, although there is a strong possibility that it may be due to a virus. It is characterised by proliferation and enlargement of the lymph nodes and spleen. Biopsy of the lymph nodes reveals the presence of large multinucleated giant cells (Reed–Sternberg cells). It occurs more commonly in males than in females. It is the commonest malignancy in young adults aged 15–34 years, although it may also occur in the elderly. The first symptom may be of an enlarged lymph node in the neck or the axilla. The disease progresses at a variable rate and initially there may be few symptoms other than night sweats, fever and weight loss.

Medical management

A combination of radiotherapy and chemotherapy has improved the survival rate, although following 'cure' of the condition, it exposes the individual to an increased risk of leukaemia. During chemotherapy patients are more susceptible to infection, oral ulceration and bleeding following surgery.

Dental care

Treatment of an invasive nature and general anaesthesia should be avoided until the patient is in remission.

Non-Hodgkin's Lymphoma

The non-Hodgkin's lymphomas (NHL) comprise a wide variety of neoplastic proliferative disorders of lymphoid cells which usually disseminate throughout the body. The characteristic cells that are present in Hodgkin's disease, notably the Reed–Sternberg cells, are absent.

These lymphomas occur in all ages, but with an increasing incidence with age and more frequently than Hodgkin's disease. Males are affected more frequently than females.

Little is known of the aetiology, which may be due to a virus. The incidence is increased following a single large dose of radiation. It may occur as a secondary malignancy in patients who have received radiation therapy and chemotherapy for a previous malignancy. There are several classifications but, in general, the greater the degree of differentiation the better the prognosis.

The initial symptoms are local or generalised enlargement of the lymph nodes which are painless. Since the tonsils are lymphoid tissue, they may also be enlarged. There may be night sweats, weight loss and anaemia.

Diagnosis is by lymph node biopsy. The prognosis depends on the degree of differentiation, but in general is not as good as with Hodgkin's disease.

Medical management

Aggressive chemotherapy and/or radiotherapy are given to induce remission. Relapse can occur due to involvement of the central nervous system (CNS), and cranial irradiation plus intrathecal methotrexate may be considered. The prognosis is poor and treatment may only be palliative. However, with some of the newer combination therapies more favourable outcomes may be possible.

Dental care

As with Hodgkin's disease, treatment should be avoided until the patient is in remission.

Effects of Radiotherapy and Chemotherapy

The early diagnosis of cancer or precancerous conditions is of the utmost importance. This may reduce the treatment necessary and may even be life saving.

The treatment and management of cancer is by surgery, and/or radiotherapy and chemotherapy, or by combinations of these. Surgery may result in the loss of some normal tissue surrounding the lesion, and if this is extensive, can lead to the loss of anatomical form and function. Treatment of cancer of the head and neck region by radiotherapy is particularly advantageous as it enables the preservation of tissue. The disadvantage of this form of treatment is that there may also be some damage to the surrounding normal or underlying tissues. Sometimes a combination of surgery and radiotherapy is indicated.

Before a patient receives radiotherapy or chemotherapy, the mouth should be fully examined, both clinically and radiographically and the prognosis of the teeth assessed. Teeth with a doubtful long-term prognosis should be extracted and other teeth restored. Efforts should be made to ensure that the periodontium is well maintained.

The main effect from radiation is that of xerostomia (dryness of the mouth and lips) as an indirect effect of irradiation of the salivary glands which results in a reduction of salivary flow. In some patients the salivary function will return to normal within a few months, in others the salivary glands will have been permanently damaged.

Salivary flow may be stimulated by the use of sugarless sweets, sorbitol-based chewing gum or methylcellulose-based saliva substitutes, all of which have varying degrees of success.

As a result of the reduction in the salivary flow

prosthetic appliances may be difficult to wear due to the lack of lubrication. There will also be a lack of the self-cleansing mechanism and a decrease in the buffering action of the saliva. An aggressive form of caries may develop which affects all surfaces of the teeth, even those smooth surfaces not normally affected.

Extractions following radiotherapy are extremely hazardous and are likely to result in osteoradionecrosis. This affects the mandible more than the maxilla as there is less collateral blood supply. If caries has resulted in exposure or infection of the pulp, efforts should be made to avoid extractions by endodontic treatment whenever possible. If extractions are unavoidable, surgery must be performed under antibiotic cover in order to reduce infection. The importance of good oral hygiene must be impressed on the patient and regular visits made to an hygienist. Daily fluoride rinses will help prevent caries.

Radiation in a child may result in arrested growth of the jaws due to damage to the growth centres (**37**). The teeth may also be affected and the extent of the damage depends on the amount of radiation and the stage of development at the time (**38**). There may be blunting of just the roots if only a small dose of radiation was given in the later stages of development, or with a greater dose there may be complete failure of development of the teeth (agenesis). Defects also occur in calcification.

Chemotherapy is the use of cytotoxic drugs that interfere with cell division and therefore suppress or reduce growth of malignant tissue. Unfortunately, there are no specific drugs which affect only malignant cells, therefore normal cells are also destroyed and in particular the bone marrow. The aim in treatment is to cause the destruction of the greatest number of malignant cells without causing damage to normal cells.

There are a large number of drugs available, and results have been improved by using a combination of drugs. Chemotherapy is most effective in the treatment of lymphoma, multiple myeloma, and the leukaemias.

Cytotoxic drugs cause a generalised suppression of the bone marrow producing leukopenia (reduction in the white blood cell count) and thrombocytopenia (reduction of platelets which results in mucosal bleeding and excessive haemorrhage following surgery). A depression of the immune response also occurs with an increased susceptibility to infection and an alteration in the inflammatory response. Once chemotherapy has been commenced it is essential that the oncologist who is supervising the patient is consulted if invasive dental treatment is necessary.

Candidal infection of the oral mucosa occurs in about 25% of patients who are immunosuppressed and it is essential that this is diagnosed and treated as soon as possible to reduce the risk of systemic candidiasis. Local treatment can be given with nystatin pastilles, amphotericin B lozenges or miconazole gel. Daily rinses with 0.12% chlorhexidine also help reduce the levels of oral candida as well as decreasing gingivitis.

Herpetic infection may also be a problem in such individuals and prophylactic treatment with acyclovir should be considered in the treatment of patients about to embark on chemotherapy.

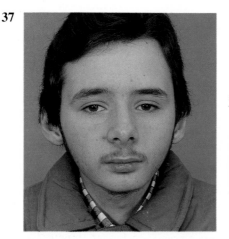

37 Radiation in this young man, who had Hodgkin's disease when he was a child, has resulted in restricted growth of the mandible due to damage to the condylar growth centres.

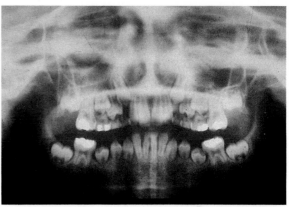

38 Orthopantomogram showing blunting of the roots of the permanent mandibular teeth as a result of radiation in that area during their development.

6 Metabolic and Endocrine Disorders

Diabetes Mellitus

Diabetes is an endocrine disorder resulting in hyperglycaemia (abnormally high blood sugar level). There may be an absolute or relative lack of insulin or the presence of factors that oppose the action of insulin.

Although diabetes has been known since ancient times, it was not until 1921 that two Canadians, Frederick Banting and Charles Best, succeeded in extracting insulin from the pancreas of dogs.

The lack of insulin causes hyperglycaemia and when this exceeds 7–12 mmol/l (the threshold level) glucose escapes into the urine (glycosuria). The presence of high levels of glucose in the bloodstream leads to an increased excretion of urine (polyuria), which eventually produces a deficit in total body water if this is not compensated for by increased fluid intake (polydipsia).

The action of insulin is to retard the release of free fatty acids from adipose tissue. In its absence there is accumulation of these free fatty acids, and neutral fat is broken down to fatty acids which are released into the bloodstream. Most of the fatty acids are oxidised to carbon dioxide and water but, when there is an excess, some of the fatty acids are converted into ketone bodies which may be detected in the urine.

Although glycosuria is nearly always indicative of diabetes, the diagnosis should be established by measuring the blood glucose, since glycosuria may occur in renal disease and pregnancy due to a fall in the renal threshold. Fasting venous whole blood/glucose levels above 7 mmol/litre of blood are diagnostic of diabetes.

Although diabetes usually occurs as a primary condition, it may occur as a result of other conditions, such as Cushing's syndrome or fibrocystic disease, and may also be caused by drugs (steroids).

There are two major forms of the condition:

- **Type I**, insulin-dependent or juvenile onset diabetes (IDDM).
- **Type II**, maturity onset diabetes – non insulin-dependent diabetes (NIDDM).

The prevalence in the UK, Western Europe and North America is about 3–4% of the population; about 10% of all diabetics have insulin-dependent diabetes mellitus. It occurs more frequently with advancing years, increasing to 20 per 1,000 in the 40–49 age group and 100 per 1,000 in those over 70 years of age. Although diabetes may occur at any age, the peak incidence for insulin-dependent diabetes is 10–12 years. The non insulin-dependent form is most common after middle-age.

There is little difference in the distribution of diabetes, though more women than men are affected, except under the age of 30 years when there is a slight male predominance.

Type I

Insulin-dependent diabetes is due to damage and eventual loss of the β cells of the pancreatic islets of Langerhans and consequent lack of insulin production. The aetiology is complex and a number of mechanisms exist, including genetic, immunological and possibly infective. Insulin-dependent diabetes is not directly inherited, although some individuals may inherit a predisposition to diabetes.

The onset of diabetes is characterised by weight loss, thirst, polyuria, polydipsia, lethargy and malaise. There may be a gradual onset and delay in diagnosis is not uncommon. Prolonged infection or the presence of candidiasis should prompt further investigation of the urine and blood.

The first aim of treatment is to control the symptoms, to prevent acute metabolic crises of ketoacidosis and hypoglycaemia and to maintain normal growth and body weight. Self reliance and self care from an early age are to be encouraged to prevent psychological complications so an optimum quality of life is achieved. To achieve an optimum life expectancy diabetic complications must be either prevented or treated early.

Thus, the blood glucose level should be kept as near to normal as possible throughout every 24 hours. This may be achieved with diet and insulin. The diet must be such that the energy requirements are met and ideal body weight achieved. There is convincing evidence to suggest that if there is good glycaemic control the development of complications is delayed or prevented.

Insulin cannot be taken by mouth because it is destroyed by the digestive processes. It therefore has to be given by injection, usually subcutaneously, except in emergencies when it should be administered intravenously. Research is proceeding with the use of an intra-nasal spray but it is difficult to achieve an accurate dosage by this means. Transplantation of a cadaveric pancreas is occasionally undertaken at the time of renal transplantation for diabetic nephropathy. Transplantation of islet cells is as yet in its infancy and is still very much experimental, but may yet prove efficacious.

Hypoglycaemia ('hypo', 'insulin reaction')

This a major hazard of insulin treatment and occurs when the blood sugar is less than 2.5 mmol/l. The symptoms, which are rapid in onset, are sweating, palpitations, shaking, tingling around the mouth, and slurred speech progressing to coma (unconsciousness). There may be difficulty in concentration and double vision. This is caused by lack of food, too little carbohydrate, extra exercise or excess insulin administration. It may be rapidly reversed by taking some form of carbohydrate, sugar or sweet drink.

All diabetics should always carry either sugar lumps, sweets or dextrasol tablets as well as identification of their diagnosis. Severe hypoglycaemia requires intravenous glucose. Prolonged severe hypoglycaemia may result in permanent brain damage.

Parents of children prone to hypoglycaemia should be taught to inject intramuscularly the hormone glucagon, which is present normally in the alpha cells of the islets of Langerhans in the pancreas, and which raises the blood glucose. Hypoglycaemia may also occur in NIDDM from excess therapy with oral hypoglycaemic drugs, e.g. sulphonylureas.

Hyperglycaemia (ketoacidosis)

This condition results from a lack of insulin and is usually due to:

- The stopping or reduction of insulin treatment, either deliberately or by mistake.
- The increased need for insulin, as a result of stress or infection.
- The onset of insulin-dependent diabetes.

Insulin treatment should never be stopped.

Early recognition of the condition is of the utmost importance. The onset of ketosis is much more gradual and the person feels thirsty, develops rapid and deep breathing and increased frequency of micturition. There may also be vomiting and abdominal pain. If insulin is not taken a diabetic coma may result.

Since hypoglycaemic coma occurs more rapidly than hyperglycaemia, a diabetic person, if found in unfamiliar surroundings, drowsy or unconscious, should be assumed to have hypoglycaemia until proved otherwise and glucose administered by whatever route is possible.

Type II

The majority of this type are usually above average weight for their height. Such patients have a relative rather than total deficiency of insulin and this may usually be controlled if their normal weight is regained and care is taken with their diet. If the diet is ineffective then oral hypoglycaemic drugs may be required.

The implications of diabetes were given by the WHO report in 1980:

- Mortality is increased twofold or threefold.
- The incidence of heart disease and strokes is greatly increased.
- Blindness is 10 times more common than in the normal population.
- Gangrene and amputation are about 20 times more common.
- Diabetes is the second leading cause of end-stage chronic renal failure.
- Other chronic disabilities may develop.

- Hospitalisation is more than twice as common as in similar age groups.
- Direct costs to medical care, for example, drugs and rehabilitation services.
- Other costs include medical services, pensions, loss of productivity and earnings due to disability.

It is important that diabetic patients are reviewed at regular intervals to assess their control, injection techniques, sites of injection and their urine and blood testing techniques. It is also advisable to have ophthalmic checks annually and priority care with chiropodists (in view of peripheral neuropathy) to give skilled care of the feet and preventive advice.

It is possible, as a diabetic person, to pursue most careers. However, there are a few exceptions, such as the armed forces, the police and drivers of long-distance and public service vehicles.

Dental care

Treatment for the well-controlled diabetic person presents few problems. The prevention of oral infection and the maintenance of healthy periodontal tissues are important. There may be accelerated periodontal breakdown in poorly controlled diabetic patients. However even in controlled diabetics there is more gingival inflammation and a significant loss of gingival attachment compared with non-diabetics. This is probably due to altered and impaired neutrophil function as neutrophils play a primary role in protection against bacterial infection. Medicines prescribed for diabetic patients should be sugar-free.

Uncontrolled diabetics have increased susceptibility to infection. Appointments should be arranged in the morning, following their insulin injection and a normal breakfast.

Local anaesthesia for restorative procedures or extractions presents no problems. General anaesthesia should never be administered to an outpatient because careful monitoring of their diabetes is necessary in order to prevent undetected hypoglycaemia during anaesthesia.

Phenylketonuria

Phenylketonuria (PKU) is a genetically determined metabolic disorder caused by a complete or near complete deficiency of phenylalanine hydroxylase. The defect is transmitted by a single recessive autosomal gene (**19**) and occurs in 1 in 10,000 to 1 in 20,000 births. Individuals with this disorder are unable to transform phenylalanine, an essential amino acid, into tyrosine. This results in excess phenylalanine circulating in the bloodstream which causes brain damage.

The baby is normal at birth but gradually becomes mentally handicapped unless diagnosed within the first few weeks of life and treated by strict dietary measures.

If untreated there is microcephaly, a prominent maxilla, widely spaced teeth and learning difficulties. Fortunately this picture is rare in countries where there is screening of the newborn. The Guthrie test is widely employed; a small amount of blood is taken around 72 hours after birth, after feeding the baby with proteins, and assayed for an elevated level of phenylalanine.

Medical management

Treatment is necessary to prevent serious mental handicap but it does not cure the condition. It is aimed at reducing the level of phenylalanine in the blood by a diet low in phenylalanine. This must be administered in the diet, as the body cannot synthesise phenylalanine. A balance must be achieved so that there is sufficient phenylalanine in the diet to maintain normal growth and development. The treatment of affected babies was pioneered by Dr Evelyn Hickman and her co-workers at the Birmingham Children's Hospital. The children had to continue with the diet into their teens, when it could be relaxed. However, there is a risk that mothers with PKU if not on a low phenylalanine diet when they become pregnant are more likely to spontaneously abort or produce babies with cardiovascular abnormalities, microcephaly and mental retardation. Prospective mothers should therefore return to a diet low in phenylalanine prior to conception.

Dental care

There may be enamel hypoplasia affecting the areas of the teeth that were calcifying at birth. The hypoplastic areas may be treated by acid-etched composite restorations or, if severe, composite or porcelain veneers.

Adrenocortical Diseases

A number of syndromes are associated with adreno-cortical insufficiency and, although uncommon, they are of importance to the dentist, as these patients may not be able to respond to infection and stress.

Primary hypoadrenalism

This occurs as a result of the inability of the adrenal glands to secrete sufficient adrenal hormones.

Addison's disease

This condition is named after Thomas Addison (1795–1860), a London physician, who first showed that the adrenal glands were essential to life.

Addison's disease, or adrenocortical insufficiency, results from the destruction of the adrenal cortex by a variety of conditions and is most commonly due to idiopathic autoimmune disease. Indeed, Addison's disease often occurs in conjunction with other auto-immune diseases, for example hypothyroidism, pernicious anaemia and insulin-dependent diabetes. Tuberculosis used to be the cause in the majority of cases in adults but now this is extremely rare. Other causes however have been identified, such as histoplasmosis, amyloidosis and metastatic tumours.

The clinical features include pigmentation, particularly of the skin and buccal mucosa, caused by the direct stimulation of adrenocorticotrophic hormone (ACTH) on the melanocytes, lassitude, muscle weakness, nausea, vomiting, and weight loss, dizziness and postural hypotension and loss of body hair. The severity of the symptoms depends upon the speed of onset of the condition and its chronicity. The most serious complication is an Addisonian crisis which may be precipitated by intercurrent illness. During an illness, increased steroids are required but in Addison's disease there is an inability to produce sufficient steroids and an acute crisis occurs with severe hypotension, dehydration and salt depletion. This constitutes a medical emergency. Diagnosis of Addison's disease is made by demonstration of adrenal insufficiency following the administration of synthetic ACTH.

Medical management

The acute condition requires urgent replacement therapy with steroids (hydrocortisone 100mg intravenously) and replacement with appropriate intravenous fluids, followed by further steroid therapy. Chronic adrenal insufficiency requires replacement therapy with adrenocortico- and mineralo-corticoids as necessary throughout life. If there is infection or stress, or if operative procedures are planned, the dose of steroids needs to be temporarily increased to prevent an adrenal crisis.

Dental care

Any patient with Addison's disease, as indeed any patient who is receiving steroid therapy or who has had steroids during the previous 12 months, requires supplemental steroids if undergoing oral surgery, and the physician supervising the administration of the steroids should be consulted. In the presence of appropriate steroid replacement therapy, there should be no effect of delayed healing nor a greater susceptibility to infection.

Secondary adrenal insufficiency

This is due to a deficiency of endogenous cortisol as a result of long-term administration of exogenous cortisol (usually prednisolone) which has caused adrenal atrophy.

Long-term steroids are prescribed for a number of conditions, including rheumatoid arthritis, severe asthma, autoimmune diseases and renal diseases (for example, nephrotic syndrome and transplantation).

Cushing's syndrome

Cushing's syndrome is a complex of symptoms and signs consequent upon a persistent and inappropriate elevation of glucocorticoid levels. It was first described by Harvey Cushing in 1932.

If precautions are not taken, the patient may develop an acute adrenal crisis. In this event, hydrocortisone (100mg) should be administered intravenously or intramuscularly and transfer arranged to a hospital.

The most common cause of Cushing's syndrome is iatrogenic, due to the administration of steroids for a number of conditions (*see* above). The next most common cause is hypersecretion of ACTH from the pituitary gland and is referred to as Cushing's disease. Over 90% of these patients have a microadenoma of the pituitary gland. Other causes of Cushing's syndrome include excess secretion of cortisol from an adrenocortical tumour, and rarely, ectopic ACTH secretion from a variety of tumours, particularly carcinoma of the bronchus or an adrenal carcinoma. Cushing's disease can occur at any age, and is more common in females, with a sex ratio of approximately 10:1.

Classically, the face is rounded and is described as 'moon face'(**39,40**). The cheeks appear prominent and flushed, giving a deceptively robust appearance. There is generalised obesity, particularly of the trunk and this has been described as a 'lemon on matchsticks'. There is a greater susceptibility to infection and poor wound healing. In children there is arrested growth and in girls there is masculinisation. Hypertension is common in all age groups, about a third of patients have associated diabetes and hypercalcuria may result in renal stones. Osteoporosis also occurs in all age groups and may result in spontaneous fractures, particularly of the axial

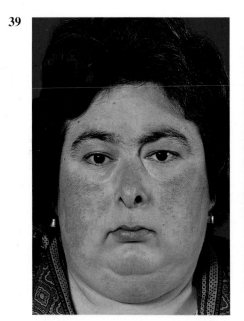

39 Classical facial features in a patient with Cushing's syndrome. 'Moon face' with prominent and flushed cheeks.

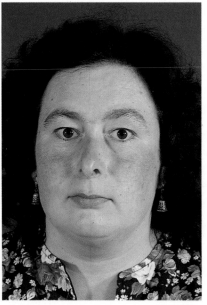

40 Patient shown in **39** following treatment.

skeleton. Following treatment in children there is healing of the bone, however, in adults, although the tendency to fracture is reduced the osteoporosis persists.

About 20% of patients suffer from depression and emotional instability. Diagnosis is made by assessing the plasma cortisol levels.

Medical management

This is to correct either the hyperfunction of the adrenal cortex or the pituitary gland, whichever is the cause. Adrenal tumours may require resection and the patient will then require steroid replacement therapy throughout life. The pituitary may require trans-sphenoidal surgery or irradiation after control has been achieved by medical therapy.

Dental care

Since patients with Cushing's syndrome are susceptible to oral infection, especially oral candidiasis, good oral hygiene is essential. However, definitive dental treatment should generally be avoided until the condition is controlled.

Thyroid Disorders

Hyperthyroidism

Hyperthyroidism, or thyrotoxicosis, results from the excessive production of thyroid hormone (T4 and/or T3). The cause of this disorder is either diffuse hyperplasia and hypertrophy, (Graves' disease), or hyperactive or 'toxic' single or multiple nodules of the thyroid gland.

It may occur at any age, more commonly in females in a ratio of 6:1, with a peak in the third and fourth decade. It is rare in children under the age of 15 years.

The appearance is characteristic, with exophthalmos (lid retraction so the sclera is visible above the iris, **41**) and an enlarged thyroid gland (goitre, **42**). The patient is agitated, restless and has a tremor. The skin is warm and moist with increased sweating and there is an intolerance to heat. Although the patient has a voracious appetite there is loss of weight. The pulse is rapid and the patient may have atrial fibrillation.

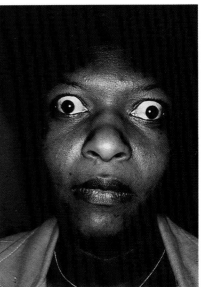

41

41 Exophthalmos in a patient with hyperthyroidism. The sclera is visible above the iris.

42

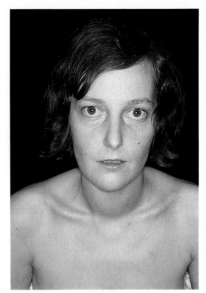

Diagnosis is usually fairly straightforward from the history and clinical picture, and it may be confirmed by assaying the level of circulating thyroid hormone T3 and T4.

42 Enlarged thyroid gland in a girl with hyperthyroidism.

Medical management

This may be medical, with the use of antithyroid drugs, usually carbimazole, and beta-adrenergic blocking agents. It must be emphasised that all drugs are not without side effects and the most dangerous side effect of carbimazole is agranulocytosis. This usually occurs within 3 months of commencing therapy and patients must be warned that they should report to their doctor urgently if they get any infection.

Regrettably, relapse occurs in over 70% of patients within 2 years and increasingly treatment with radio-active iodine is being used as first line therapy in view of its relative safety, although there is an increased incidence of subsequently developing hypothyroidism.

If the thyroid gland is very enlarged and if it is causing compression of adjacent structures, then surgical management is indicated. Prior to surgery, the patient must be made euthyroid by medical therapy. Surgery, too, is not without side effects, as it may result in injury to the recurrent laryngeal nerve and cause hoarseness.

Dental care

This should be avoided until the patient's condition is controlled.

Hypothyroidism

Hypothyroidism (myxoedema) results from a deficiency of thyroid hormone. It may become apparent during the first few weeks of life and may be due to aplasia or hypoplasia of the thyroid gland. It is essential that new-born babies are screened, as delay in diagnosis results in retardation of physical, but perhaps more importantly, mental, development. Hypothyroidism in children is named cretinism (from the French crétien, meaning Christian, as such children appeared very meek and mild). Affected children have depression of the bridge of the nose, narrow slanted eyes with swollen lids, and protrusion of an enlarged tongue through an open mouth. The baby sleeps a lot, is a poor feeder and may suffer from respiratory distress.

In adults, hypothyroidism is either secondary to an autoimmune disease or a result of treatment for hyperthyroidism.

The onset is often insidious, the skin is dry, coarse and scaly. There is puffiness and periorbital swelling (**43**). There is loss of hair and an increase in weight. The patient is slow, lethargic and forgetful. There is macroglossia and speech may be affected, this has been described as a gruff voice like a gramophone running down. There is enlargement of the heart and bradycardia. The diagnosis is made by measurement of the levels of thyroxine.

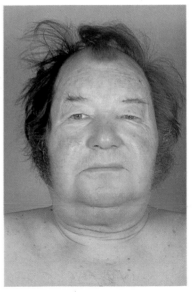

Medical management

Replacement therapy with thyroxine.

Dental care

There should be no problems with dental treatment in a patient under control with thyroxine unless there are cardiac complications.

43 Patient with myxoedema, the eyelids are swollen and the eyes appear narrowed. There is also an increase in weight.

Parathyroid Disorders

Hypoparathyroidism

There may be congenital absence of the glands (DiGeorge syndrome), in which there are gross immunological deficiencies, midline clefts, micrognathia and hypertelorism. There may be mental retardation and hypocalcaemia which can cause major convulsions and tetany. Death usually occurs in early childhood.

Hypoparathyroidism may also result from damage to the glands during surgery of the thyroid glands or it may be idiopathic. Diagnosis is made by assessing the levels of serum calcium and parathormone.

If hypoparathyroidism occurs in adults, the radiographic appearance may show a generalised alteration of the trabecular pattern, resulting in a 'ground glass' appearance. There may be accompanying loss of the lamina dura around the teeth. However, this is not a consistent finding as has often been stated in the past. Brown tumours may also occur in the jaws and may be seen on radiographs as either unilocular or multilocular radiolucencies.

Medical management

Appropriate replacement therapy, usually with 1-alpha hydroxycholecalciferol.

Dental care

Candidiasis may be a problem. The teeth may be hypoplastic if the condition was due to congenital absence of glands. In adults the radiographic radiolucencies may be due to brown tumours.

7 Gastroenterological Disorders

Coeliac Disease (Gluten-Induced Enteropathy)

The first mention of this condition was in the second half of the second century AD by Galen, a Roman physician. The Greek word 'koiliakos' means 'suffering in the bowels'.

In 1950 Professor Dicke, a Dutch paediatrician, showed how coeliac children improved dramatically when wheat, rye and oat flour were excluded from their diet. Replacement with maize or rice flour resulted in absorption of fat and an improvement in appetite and general health.

Coeliac disease is a disorder of the small intestine caused by intolerance to the gliadin fraction of gluten which is one of the protein fractions of wheat, barley, rye and oats. It occurs in 0.1% of the population and there seems to be a familial predisposition suggesting a genetic basis. It is probably inherited as an autosomal dominant trait with incomplete expressivity. It is characterised by degenerative changes in the mucosa (villous dystrophia). It results in a chronic malabsorption disorder with abdominal distension, pale, bulky, foul smelling stools, wasting of muscles, anaemia and retarded growth and weight gain.

Diagnosis can be confirmed by a biopsy of the jejunum which shows flattened mucosa with lack of villi therefore resulting in malabsorption. The villi return to normal following elimination of gluten from the diet.

Symptoms of diarrhoea, abdominal discomfort and nutritional deficiencies may occur in a baby with the introduction of mixed feeding; but the diagnosis may be delayed for several years until adult life, when mild chronic ill health may be the only symptom. Clinically the condition ranges from near normal health to severe intestinal malabsorption.

Medical management

All gluten-containing food must be avoided and this results in a return to normal of the intestinal mucosa and a dramatic improvement in general health and well being. A gluten-free diet requires longer to prepare and many convenience foods must be avoided owing to the presence of wheat flour. This special diet is recommended throughout life. Booklets are available through the Coeliac Society which list gluten-free products available.

Dental care

Hypoplasia of the permanent dentition may occur in those teeth forming at the time solids were first introduced into the diet. The severity of the hypoplasia probably depends on the severity of the condition and

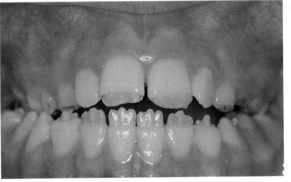

44 Chronological hypoplasia affecting the permanent dentition in a patient with coeliac disease. The permanent upper and lower central incisors and the lower lateral incisors and canines are affected as these teeth were forming when the patient commenced mixed feeding (on weaning). Following diagnosis, with dietary control, calcification has proceeded normally. Note that the upper lateral incisor teeth have escaped this hypoplasia due to their later development.

the time that elapsed between the onset of symptoms and the initiation of treatment (**44**). The defects can usually be treated by acid-etch composite restorations.

Apthous ulceration of the oral mucosa is common and responds to a gluten-free diet. In general, dental treatment does not present any problems.

Crohn's Disease

Crohn's disease is a chronic recurrent inflammatory disease affecting the alimentary tract which causes major disability, mostly in young people. The condition was first highlighted by Crohn, Ginzburg and Oppenheimer in 1932 but descriptions of the disease had been published by others before that time.

The aetiology of Crohn's disease is uncertain but it seems to occur more frequently in Western populations and particularly affects the Jewish race. It occurs most commonly in young adults and there is no sex difference in the incidence.

Inflammatory changes in the ileo-caecal region are most common, giving rise to abdominal pain and malabsorption. Oral lesions occur in around 6–20% of patients and include ulcers, labial and facial swelling, mucosal 'tags' or 'cobblestones' and proliferation of the oral mucosa.

Medical management

There is no specific therapy and a wide range of treatment has been tried. Elemental diets may relieve the symptoms in some. (Elemental diets were developed in the 1960s for astronauts to solve the problems of storage, ingestion and waste disposal. They are composed of amino acids and small peptides as the nitrogen source, with up to 30% of energy supplied as fat. There is no lactose or digestive residues, and trace metals and vitamins are added to the recommended daily requirement.) Antibiotics are necessary if there are fistulae or infection, corticosteroids may be beneficial in the acute stages and immunosuppressive drugs have produced some dramatic results. If medical treatment is not successful, surgery may be necessary, particularly to treat bowel stenoses or fistulae.

Dental care

45

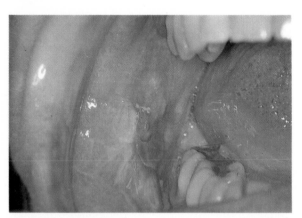

Oral lesions may be the first indication of the disease and the patient should be referred to a gastroenterologist for further investigation (**45**).

45 'Cobblestone' appearance of the buccal mucosa in a patient with Crohn's disease.

Ulcerative Colitis

Although there is no proof of the cause of ulcerative colitis it appears to represent a heterogenous group of conditions caused by multiple environmental factors.

About 4–20% of patients with ulcerative colitis have recurrent apthous ulcerations. They may also have diffuse swellings of the cheeks and lips, chronic hyperplasia and a cobblestone appearance of the mucosa and hyperplastic gingivitis (*see* **45**).

Medical management.

Sulphasalazine may aid the induction and maintenance of remission. Occasionally there is spontaneous remission. Topical or systemic steroids may also be of value.

Dental care

Oral lesions may respond when the symptoms of colitis are treated medically or surgically.

8 Chromosomal Disorders

Down's Syndrome (Trisomy 21)

Down's syndrome is a genetic condition and is the commonest cause of retardation of mental development. Although the condition has been known for many centuries it was not until 1866 that it was formally described by an English physician, John Langdon Down.

The incidence in the UK is 1.5 per 1,000 births. The majority of those with Down's syndrome have three of the chromosome 21 (trisomy 21), which occurs as a result of chromosomal non-dysjunction, thus there is a total of 47 chromosomes instead of the normal 46. However 5% of those with Down's syndrome have a different kind of chromosome mutation called translocation, in which only part of chromosome 21 is present in triplicate. This occurs when a piece of chromosome 21 attaches itself most often to chromosome 13, 14, 15, 21 or 22.

It is important to know which type is involved, as where there is translocation, further children are likely to be affected. Trisomy is more common in older mothers; over 40 years of age the incidence rises to 1 in 50 and over 45 years to 1 in 20 births. Women over the age of 35 years should be informed of the risk of producing a baby with Down's syndrome so that amniocentesis or chorionic villus biopsy may be offered early in pregnancy to exclude the condition.

Over 20% of babies with Down's syndrome are born to mothers over 35 years old, yet these older mothers account for only approximately 6% of the total births. However, in recent years there does seem to have been an increase in the number of women over the age of 35 years having babies.

Down's syndrome is a generalised defect and affects most tissues. In appearance those affected resemble each other (**46**): they have a brachycephalic skull and there may be delayed closure of the fontanelles.

There is a generalised defect in growth, particularly in endochondral ossification, resulting in reduction in their average height. The defective growth at the spheno-occipital synchondrosis and the sphenomaxillary suture results in underdevelopment of the middle third of the face. This gives the appearance of mandibular prognathism.

The eyes are slanting and have prominent epicanthic folds. The iris in babies may show a spotted appearance (Brushfield's spots).

The tongue is relatively large, fissured and tends to protrude (**47,48**). The hands are short and the little finger turns inwards (**49**), and there may also be a deep transverse crease across the palm (simian crease).

Physical development is delayed and after puberty there is a tendency to adiposity. Advice regarding healthy eating and the avoidance of snacks should be given in childhood and adolescence. Speech is delayed and may be defective with a husky, low pitched voice.

Cardiovascular lesions are present in about 40–50% of those with Down's syndrome and may be the cause of early death (**50–53**). About 10% have

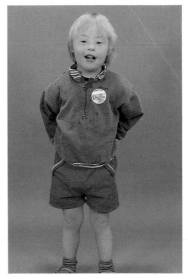

46

46 A 3-year-old boy with Down's syndrome showing the typical facial features.

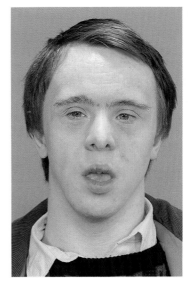

47

47 Boy with Down's syndrome. Note the dry scaly skin and enlarged and protrusive tongue.

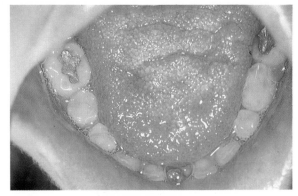

48 Enlarged and fissured tongue in Down's syndrome.

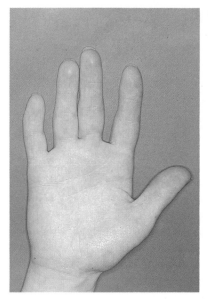

49 The hand is short and square and the little finger turns inwards in Down's syndrome.

epilepsy, there is an increased incidence of cataracts, and also an increased incidence of leukaemia, which is usually the acute lymphoblastic type. More recently a genetic link has been discovered between Down's syndrome and Alzheimer's disease.

People with Down's Syndrome are also susceptible to respiratory infections, they may have hearing deficiency, the skin is rather dry and scaly, and frequently they have eczema.Those living in institutions have a higher risk of carrying hepatitis B virus (HBsAg).

The degree of intellectual impairment varies widely but intelligence rarely reaches the mental age of 7 years. The intelligence quotient (IQ) is in the range of 20–80 with an average of about 50.

They interact better socially than other people who have similar learning difficulties. They are fond of music and have a loving personality as children but as they grow older they may become aggressive and somewhat stubborn.

In Down's syndrome, the teeth may be delayed in development and therefore be delayed in eruption. The teeth are usually smaller than normal and there may be congenital absence of teeth (hypodontia), usually the upper lateral incisors.

The caries incidence is about the same as the average, but there is a higher incidence of periodontal disease with progressive loss of the supporting bone, particularly affecting the lower incisors. Although oral hygiene may be poor, the severity of the periodontal disease is much greater than in people with equivalent oral hygiene; this may be due to an immunological deficiency and/or a metabolic block in collagen maturation.

Malocclusions occur as a result of the under-development of the maxilla and failure to grow downwards and forwards. A Class III incisor relationship occurs in about a third of individuals and the enlarged tongue often results in an anterior open bite and a posterior cross-bite.

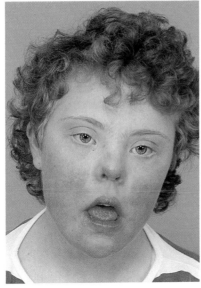

50 Girl with Down's syndrome and associated Fallot's tetralogy which was considered to be inoperable. She has cyanosis affecting all tissues.

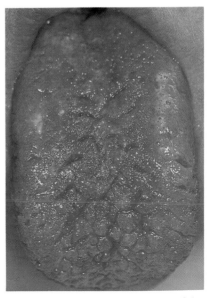

51 Fissured and cyanotic tongue of the girl in **50**.

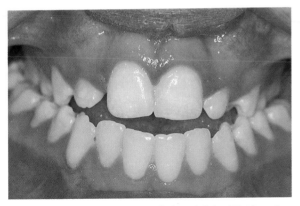

52 Intra-oral appearance of the girl in **50** showing cyanosis of the oral tissues.

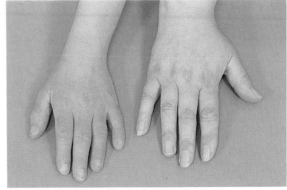

53 The hand on the left is that of the girl shown in **50**. The cyanosis is obvious when compared with her mother's hand on the right.

Dental care

If the patient has a heart defect, antibiotics must be given prior to procedures likely to cause a bacteraemia. Pulp treatments in the primary teeth are contraindicated. Endodontic treatment may be considered in the permanent anterior teeth if an adequate apical seal can be obtained.

Chlorhexidine gels or mouthwashes may be of some help in controlling the periodontal disease. Orthodontic treatment may not be possible due to the skeletal discrepancy, and co-operation problems.

Dentures should be considered if there are missing anterior teeth. The degree of co-operation for dental treatment is related largely to the level of intelligence. The patient requires a confident, sympathetic and caring approach.

If there are severe learning difficulties a general anaesthetic may be necessary in order to carry out dental treatment.

Prader–Willi Syndrome

The Prader–Willi syndrome is a complex medical condition with multiple handicaps and was first described by Professor Prader (a Swiss Paediatric endocrinologist), Professor Labhart (a professor of medicine), and Dr Willi (a physician) in 1956. In the seventeenth century a Spanish artist Juan Correno de Mirada who painted two portraits of a girl with this condition.

The true incidence is not known but about 1 in 40,000 of the population is affected world-wide. Boys and girls are equally affected but the condition is usually found in only one member of a family.

At birth the baby appears floppy and has difficulty suckling as a result of hypotonia of the muscles. Usually at about the age of 2–4 years the child develops an insatiable appetite which is probably due to an abnormality in the hypothalamus. If not controlled, gross obesity results (**54**) and death may occur due to cardiopulmonary insufficiency. There may be learning difficulties, lack of normal sexual development and maturity and emotional instability. Diabetes may be an added complication.

The face has a characteristic appearance with a high forehead, almond-shaped eyes and a prominent nasal bridge (**55**). Sexual development is usually minimal. Affected persons have a similar personality to those people with Down's syndrome — warm, friendly and loving, but there may be outbursts of temper. The basic defect appears to be in the hypothalamus.

The main problem is the voracious appetite and consequent obesity. There is a lowered IQ, continuous care and support is necessary throughout life and independence is rarely achieved.

54

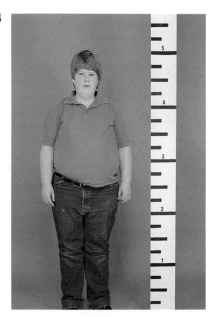

55

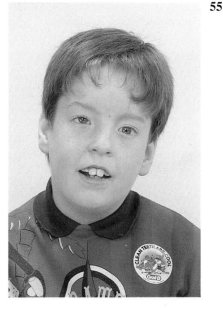

54 A 14-year-old boy with Prader–Willi syndrome. He is obese due to his voracious appetite, caused by this condition.

55 Typical facial features of Prader–Willi syndrome in a 5-year-old boy. Note the almond-shaped eyes and high forehead.

Medical management

Various drugs have been used in an attempt to control the appetite but with little success. Once the patient has become obese, weight reduction is virtually impossible.

Dental care

As a result of the constant intake of food and drink there may be a higher incidence of caries and erosion may also be a feature (**56–58**).

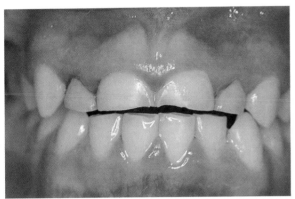

56 Intra-oral view of boy in **54** showing a combination of attrition and erosion of his permanent incisor teeth.

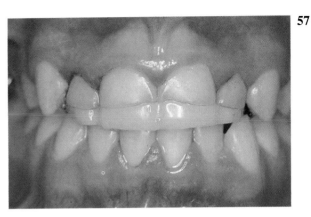

57 Appliance used to open the bite anteriorly in order to restore the permanent incisor teeth (same patient as **54**).

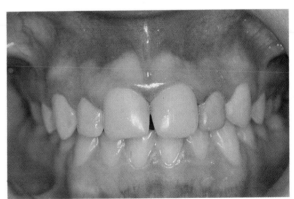

58 Composite restorations placed to restore the dimensions of the permanent incisor teeth (same patient as **54**).

There are numerous complex syndromes, mostly of unknown aetiology, with defects of the genes and mental abnormalities. When treating these patients it is helpful to know about their disabilities but also their capabilities. One such example is the Rubinstein–Taybi syndrome.

Rubinstein–Taybi Syndrome

Rubinstein–Taybi syndrome occurs sporadically in otherwise normal families and is of unknown aetiology. There is retardation of growth, low set ears and abnormalities of the hands and feet (**59,60**). There are moderate to severe learning difficulties and they are unlikely to be able to achieve independent existence.

59

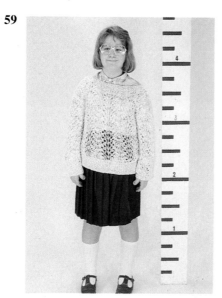

59 A 14-year-old girl with Rubinstein–Taybi syndrome.

60

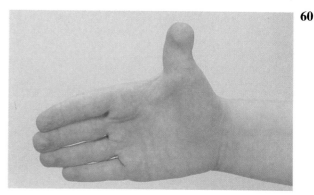

60 Abnormal thumb joint of the girl in **59**.

Dental care

This depends on the degree of co-operation that can be achieved.

9 Neurological Disorders

Hydrocephalus

Hydrocephalus occurs as a result of imbalance between the production and absorption of cerebrospinal fluid. The raised pressure results in irreversible enlargement of the cranium. The circumference of the head may be normal at birth but then may grow rapidly. This may be due to congenital stenosis of the aqueduct of Sylvius. It is essential to make serial measurements of the head circumference if hydrocephalus is suspected. Skull X-rays and computerised tomography may also be necessary to confirm the diagnosis.

Medical management.

The outlook and treatment of hydrocephalus in children has improved dramatically with the introduction of the Spitz–Holter valve in 1958. The obstruction is bypassed or the excess fluid is shunted off elsewhere in the body, usually into the peritoneum (ventriculo-peritoneal shunt) (61,62), although shunts into the atrium (ventriculo-atrial) have also been used. Shunts have to be carefully maintained throughout life because they may become blocked as a result of raised protein in the cerebrospinal fluid or bacterial colonisation, resulting in immune-complex nephritis.

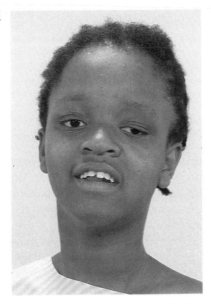

61 Girl with hydrocephalus who has had the obstruction bypassed by a shunt, thereby preventing gross enlargement of the cranium (*see* **62**).

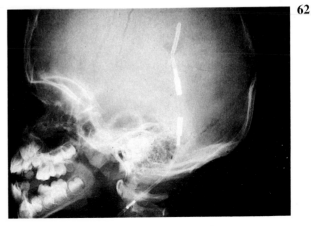

62 Lateral skull radiograph or 'shuntogram' showing the shunt.

Dental care

Since there is a danger that a bacteraemia may cause blockage of the shunt and acute renal failure, antibiotic cover is essential for any invasive dental treatment.

Spina Bifida

Spina bifida is caused by defective closure of the vertebral column in the lumbosacral region due to a defect of skin, vertebral arches and neural tube. The severity varies from a completely open spine (rachischisis) which is not usually compatible with life, to a defect in the vertebral column with a sac containing meninges (meningocoele), spinal cord (myelocoele), or both (myelomeningocoele). Indeed, minor defects in the vertebral column (spina lumbosacral occulta) may be present in the absence of neurological signs. Paralysis occurs below the level of involvement. There may be complete paralysis of the lower limbs and the sphincters of the bladder and rectum. There may also be a club foot or dislocated hip.

Diagnosis can be made *in utero* using amniocentesis to detect an elevation in the α-feto protein (APF) and acetylcholinesterase. The incidence is 0.2–4% of the population and is higher in females. The incidence varies in different parts of the world, with an increased incidence in the Welsh and Irish. Nutritional factors, particularly vitamin deficiencies, have been suggested as a possible cause.

Recent evidence has shown that hydrocephalus may be due to folate deficiency and that giving folate to those expectant mothers who may be at risk has resulted in a reduced incidence.

Medical management.

Early closure of the defect is necessary to prevent infection. There may also be associated hydrocephalus which necessitates the insertion of a shunt. The prognosis depends on the amount of motor involvement and the severity of other abnormalities.

Dental care

Prophylactic antibiotics are necessary in the presence of a shunt.

Cerebral Palsy

Cerebral palsy was described by Dr W.J. Little in 1853. 'Cerebral' means brain and 'palsy' means impairment. It is a non-progressive lesion of the brain resulting in impairment and incoordination of the muscles. It is one of the commonest physical handicapping conditions in children and affects about 2 per 1,000 school age children. Males are more commonly affected than females. About 40% have some degree of mental retardation.

Cerebral palsy may result from anything which can cause damage to the brain either pre-natally, such as maternal viral infection, peri-natally, as a result of cerebral anoxia, or post-natally, as a result of meningitis, trauma to the head or kernicterous due to rhesus incompatibility. Its cause, however, may be difficult to ascertain.

There is a wide range in the degree of involvement. There are some who are affected only minimally, while others are so severely affected that continuous hospital care is necessary. Classification of the condition is based on the motor involvement.

Spastic cerebral palsy

This is the most common form, affecting about half of those with cerebral palsy. There is increased activity of the deep tendons and the muscles feel stiff and rigid. This form is due to damage to the cortex of the brain and it may be classified according to the extent of the involvement:

- Hemiplegia accounts for about a third of those affected.
- Diplegia. All the limbs are involved but the lower limbs are more severely affected.

- Paraplegia. Only the lower limbs are affected.
- Quadriplegia. All the limbs are affected and there is usually mental handicap and epilepsy as well (**63,64**).

63

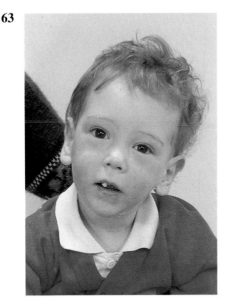

64

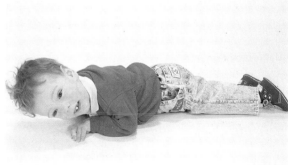

63,64 A 3-year-old boy with quadraplegic cerebral palsy.

Athetoid cerebral palsy

In this form of cerebral palsy there is hypotonia in early infancy followed by athetoid movements in later childhood. It is due to damage of the basal ganglion and is usually caused by severe jaundice in the neonatal period (kernicterous) and can be prevented by appropriate treatment of hyperbilirubinaemia.

Muscles contract involuntarily resulting in twisting and contorted movements (**65,66**).

Speech may also be affected as a result of abnormal movements of the tongue and vocal cords. Speech defects may give a misleading impression of the intelligence and although the patient may fully understand what is said, he or she may have difficulty in being understood, thus leading to communication difficulties. The more severely affected individuals may need aids to enable them to communicate. Symbols were devised by Charles K. Bliss in the 1940s as a possible international language. These are pictographs and symbols which are displayed on a chart and can be pointed to by a finger, eye, head pointer or even by an electronic device.

65   **66**

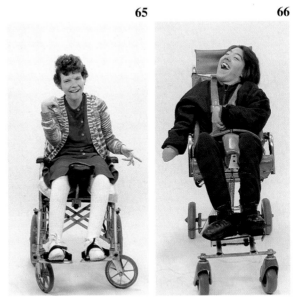

65,66 Two girls with athetoid cerebral palsy. They have involuntary, writhing, and contorted movements.

Ataxic cerebral palsy

This form is due to injury to the cerebellum and results in an unsteady gait and difficulty in balance control. Again speech is usually affected and epilepsy commonly occurs.

Management

When cerebral palsy is diagnosed, parents may have a feeling of guilt or resentment and are often over-protective. A positive approach is essential in the management of people with all forms of cerebral palsy, with emphasis on what they can do rather than what they are unable to do.

Those people who are confined to a wheelchair may have a problem in weight control. Advice regarding diet is essential since weight loss is difficult to achieve and those who are overweight place an added strain on their carers.

A problem that causes great concern is that of

constant drooling and this occurs in about 10% of children. It results from the abnormal increased tone of the oral musculature, maintaining the mouth in an open position. Saliva is not swallowed and drains or dribbles on to the chin and neck resulting in maceration of the skin and this may even cause fluid depletion and dehydration. Some improvement has been achieved in those with severe problems, by relocating the mandibular salivary gland duct to the tonsillar region.

The outlook for a child with cerebral palsy largely depends on the severity of the condition and the associated mental state. Great changes have taken place in recent years regarding their treatment. In 1950 Dr Andreas Peto established the Institute of Kinesitherapy in Budapest, Hungary. The furniture at the Institute is extremely simple, consisting only of a plinth on which the children do their exercises, this is covered by a plastic cloth at meal times, and at night becomes a bed (**67**).

The objects are to help children to develop in all ways and to achieve as much independence as possible without the aid of wheelchairs. The conductors, who are teachers or special educators are responsible for all the children's requirements, emotional, cognitive and academic. Results from Hungary have been encouraging in certain types of cerebral palsy and centres are now being established in other parts of the world.

67

67 A 3-year-old being instructed in toothbrushing at a conductive education unit. Note the simple, slatted furniture.

Oral problems

Oral hygiene may be difficult for the patient and their carers. Chewing can be difficult and many cerebral palsy patients are on a soft diet. There is poor muscular control and the self-cleansing mechanism may not be very effective thus allowing the accumulation of plaque and calculus with resultant gingival inflammation.

Surveys have shown a higher number of decayed,

missing or filled teeth (DMF) than normal, specifically there are more carious and extracted teeth than in a comparable group without cerebral palsy.

There is a high incidence of teeth clenching and bruxism resulting in marked attrition with additional erosive features (*see* page 115). In some patients there is enamel hypoplasia that may be related to the episode which resulted in cerebral palsy. There is a higher incidence of traumatised incisor teeth, due to frequent falls. There may be an anterior open bite, high arched palate and malocclusion because of the abnormal muscular pattern (**68**).

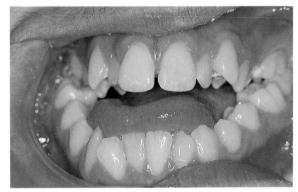

68 Anterior open bite and high arched palate of the girl in **66.**

Dental care

Many patients have specially adapted wheelchairs which give them support and it may be better to treat them in their own chair. This is possible using a special base into which the wheelchair fits (**69**). These are expensive items of equipment and an alternative may be the use of a bean bag in the dental chair moulded around the patient to give support.

There may be irregular movements of the head and body, making treatment difficult. Indeed, with the athetoid form excessive stress results in increased body movements. The more the patient tries to assist the worse the movements become.

There is a wide variation in the severity of the condition and also in the acceptance of treatment; it is usually sensible to restrict treatment to short visits in view of the short attention span.

A stainless steel mouth mirror and a finger guard,

such as a thimble, may be necessary in order to protect both the patient and the operator.

Toothbrushing may be difficult and adaptations to the toothbrush can be made to improve the grip (**70**). Electric toothbrushes and regular visits to a hygienist may both be beneficial.

Treatment of the teeth in the anterior part of the mouth may not present too much of a problem. However restorations on the posterior teeth can be difficult due to the bite reflex.

Although orthodontic treatment is possible, in some patients it may result in an unstable position of the teeth, necessitating permanent retention. In some patients, restorative treatment may not be possible without a general anaesthetic and this is best carried out under 'day stay' conditions.

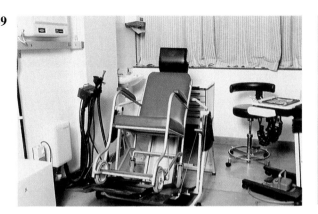

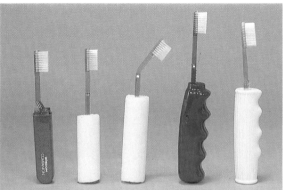

69 Specially constructed wheelchair base which enables the patient to be reclined for dental treatment in their own wheelchair (courtesy of Dr A.S.T. Franks).

70 Toothbrushes with various adaptations to improve the grip (courtesy of Dr A.S.T. Franks).

Multiple Sclerosis

Multiple sclerosis (MS, disseminated sclerosis) is a chronic degenerative disease affecting the central nervous system. It affects the myelin or white matter of the brain and spinal cord.

It was first described by a French pathologist, Jean Cruveilhier, in 1930, and later by Sir Robert Carswell, a Scottish physician and pathologist. Three distinct signs were described by Jean-Martin Charcot, nystagmus, intention tremor and scanning speech, and these are known as Charcot's triad.

It rarely occurs in childhood, the usual age of onset being between 20 and 40 years of age, and is slightly more common in females. The cause is unknown but it often affects fit and healthy young people. Many theories have been put forward, including 'slow' viruses, immunological mechanisms, and deficiencies of essential fatty acids.

There is demyelination of the myelin sheath with resultant motor and sensory dysfunction. Initial symptoms may be excessive fatigue, loss of vision, diplopia, and ataxia. Intellectual ability is not usually affected in the early stages but there may be dementia in advanced disease.

Diagnosis is often difficult due to the wide range of symptoms. The condition is characterised by multiple lesions in space and time with acute attacks and remissions. Following remissions, there may not be a complete return to the previous healthy state. It has been likened to bouncing a ball at the top of a staircase. The ball may bounce up and down on the same stair but eventually it moves down to the next stair and so on down the staircase.

In some patients there may only be one attack and complete return to normal, in others just a few exacerbations with symptom-free intervals, but there may not be a complete return to normal. Alternatively there may be a gradual deterioration with increasing disability and ultimate confinement to a wheelchair.

Examination by magnetic resonance imaging (MRI) may show evidence of plaques in the brain.

Medical management

Drugs to relieve symptoms are given on an empirical basis. Corticosteroids (prednisone, 60mg /day for 5 days) may be effective in acute exacerbations, but long-term they lose their efficacy and produce undesirable side effects.

Patients should be dissuaded from chasing after 'cures' such as the replacement of amalgam restorations.

Weight control is important as with any patient who may become wheelchair bound.

Dental care

Infection should be avoided as it may exacerbate the condition.

Short appointments are necessary as muscle weakness may limit the time the patient can keep his or her mouth open. Ataxia and poor co-ordination may cause difficulties in using a mouthwash. Patients may suffer from vertigo which is made worse when placed in a supine position. As many patients may be wheelchair bound and have loss of co-ordination, extra support may be necessary during treatment. It is essential to have toilet facilities which have access for wheelchairs, as patients with multiple sclerosis have poor bladder control.

Tuberous Sclerosis

Tuberous sclerosis (Bournville disease) is a neuro-cutaneous syndrome and a major cause of mental defect. It is inherited as an autosomal dominant trait (**16**) and the condition ranges from mild to severe. Convulsions may commence in infancy and occur in about 90% of patients. There may also be behavioural disturbances and hyperactivity. Pigmented skin lesions occur affecting the arms, legs and body, and adenoma sebaceum occurs in a 'butterfly' distribution on the face (**71**).

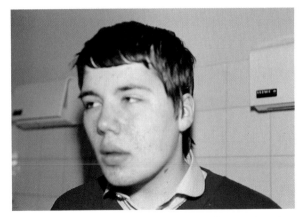

71 A 14-year-old boy with severe epilepsy showing classical 'butterfly' distribution of adenoma sebaceum associated with tuberous sclerosis.

Medical management

This is concerned with management of the convulsions and control of the hyperactivity. The prognosis depends on the severity of the condition and in severe cases death may occur as a result of status epilepticus or a brain tumour.

Dental care

This must involve maintenance of the dentition. If co-operation cannot be achieved a general anaesthetic under 'day stay' conditions may be necessary.

Epilepsy

The term 'epilepsy' comes from the Greek and means a seizure. Epilepsy is not a disease but a symptom of an underlying brain disorder. It may occur as a result of injury at birth, from hypoglycaemia (excess insulin), anoxia, cerebral tumours, toxins, trauma, sunstroke, metabolic or endocrine disorders or severe hypotension.

Seizures or convulsions are more common in infants because the nervous system is immature and therefore more unstable. They occur with a sudden rise in temperature (pyrexia) and are common with pneumonia, otitis media and the exanthemata, so called febrile convulsions.

Epilepsy affects about 0.5–1.0% of the population and commonly occurs in mentally, physically or multiply handicapped people but only 5% of epileptics are mentally handicapped. It can occur at any age but more than 70% have their first attack before the age of 20 years. In teenagers and young adults epilepsy is usually idiopathic while over the age of 40 years structural or metabolic causes are more common. In the majority of patients no cause can be established. There may be only a slight twitch or there may be loss of consciousness.

Petit mal seizures

There is a transient loss of consciousness and an upward rolling of the eyes. This condition may disappear at around puberty. If the child is doing something, he or she will discontinue and then resume when the seizure has ended as though nothing has happened.

A seizure may occur as a result of hyperventilation or a flashing light of a certain frequency, such as occurs at discotheques.

Post-traumatic epilepsy may occur following head injuries. The attacks may start several days after the trauma. In order to prevent this, it may be advisable for patients who have received such a trauma to have a course of anticonvulsant drugs.

Grand mal seizures

These are usually preceded by a warning (aura) which is followed by tonic and then clonic convulsions and loss of consciousness. The patient falls and may develop laryngeal spasm resulting in cyanosis. The spasm of the masticatory muscles may result in the patient biting the lip or tongue. Incontinence may occur. The patient usually awakes with a headache and in a state of confusion.

Medical management

This is aimed at reducing and preventing further attacks. Various anticonvulsant drugs are available and the dose should be sufficient to control the seizures but not so excessive as to cause oversedation.

If the attacks are not controlled there may be mental deterioration. There are a number of anticonvulsant drugs available, including phenobarbitone, phenytoin, carbamazepine, sodium valproate and primidone. Two newer drugs, vigabatrin and lamotrigine, await further evaluation as to their long-term efficacy. Diazepam is not suitable as an anticonvulsant but may be used in a patient with status epilepticus (seizures occurring continuously without remission). If recurrent attacks occur then sedation with chlormethiazole is employed and if this is ineffective, paralysis and ventilation may be necessary until the attack abates.

There have been a number of surveys which show that there is an increased incidence of congenital malformations in babies born to women with epilepsy. This may be due to the drugs which the mother is taking. However, if the mother ceases to take the drugs there is a risk that her fits may result in fetal anoxia.

Trauma may result in fractures of the facial skeleton, and severe uncontrolled epileptics may need to wear protective headgear to avoid damage to the cranium (**72**).

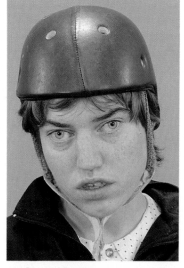

72

72 Girl who has uncontrolled epilepsy wearing protective headgear.

Dental care

Fractures of the teeth are a common occurrence (**73**). In patients whose epilepsy is well controlled and who are not mentally handicapped, treatment of these injuries presents no added problems. Where there is lack of co-operation due to learning difficulties or multiple handicaps a general anaesthetic may be necessary. If a tooth has been avulsed re-implantation is not advisable. However, there is no contra-indication for replacement of missing teeth with dentures if these are adequately retained with clasps. Although phenytoin is effective in controlling seizures, it results in gingival hyperplasia in about 50% of patients. In some patients the gingival hyperplasia can be controlled by good oral hygiene (**74,75**). In others, the hyperplasia is so severe that it may prevent the eruption of the teeth (**76**). In patients where there is excessive hyperplasia, there should be discussion with the patient's doctor to see if the drug could be changed. A gingivectomy may be necessary to improve the appearance but if the drug is not changed and if oral hygiene is not maintained to a very high standard then hyperplasia will recur.

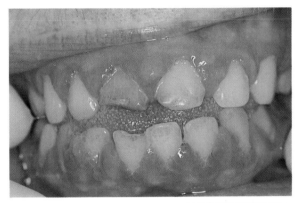

73 Intra-oral view of girl in **72** showing gingival hyperplasia and previous traumatic injuries to the permanent anterior teeth which have occurred during fits.

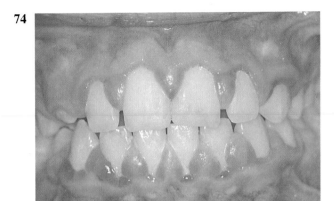

74 Gingival hyperplasia in a girl who is epileptic and taking phenytoin.

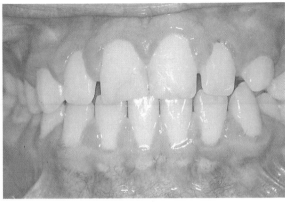

75 Patient shown in **74** several weeks after she had received a scale and polish and advice regarding toothbrushing. There is still some residual hyperplasia, but there has been a marked improvement in her gingival health.

Seizures may occur following a general anaesthetic and patients require supervision for several hours post-operatively. Seizures may also occur in the dental chair and it is important to protect the patients from harming either themselves or the equipment.

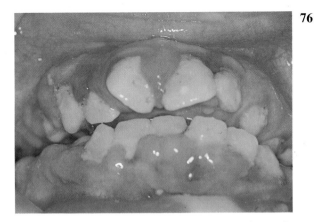

76 Severe form of hyperplasia in a patient on phenytoin who also has problems related to her oral hygiene.

Autism

Autism was first described by an American child psychiatrist, Leo Kanner, in 1944. Autistic children look physically normal and may have normal or even superior intelligence but are frequently mistaken as being mentally handicapped. Autism is a comparatively rare condition affecting 0.7–4.5 in 1,000 children and is more common in males in the ratio 4:1. The term 'autism' is derived from the Greek 'autos', meaning self. There is a profound inability to relate to people, with extreme aloneness and withdrawal and apparent disconnection from the world around. There is an obsessive desire for sameness.

There are severe defects in speech development and there is a form of language which is difficult to interpret, this may be the reason for referral. Tests must be performed to exclude deafness. In some instances the condition may go undiagnosed until the age of 4 or 5 years.

Usually the parents have been aware of a lack of response from the baby and there may be an absence of smiling. Indeed, the baby may become rigid when held, turn away and cannot be consoled. Parents find this indifference and hostility extremely difficult to accept, it is quite unlike the children with Down's syndrome who are loving and responsive. Autistic children are unable to form emotional relationships and there is sometimes an affectionate relationship with an inanimate object. Objects seem safer to relate to than people.

Autistic children develop rituals that cannot be broken and they may become fixed or obsessed by one object. Changes in routine may result in intense disturbance and temper tantrums. Tantrums and anti-social behaviour are thought not to be attention seeking, rather due to an expression of inner confusion, fear and frustration. Eye contact may be impossible to achieve and there may be head banging and grinding of the teeth. There may also be holding of food in the mouth, refusal of solid foods and insistence of soft foods. Many autistic children are hyperactive.

Medical management

Many forms of treatment have been tried. Drugs such as the beta-blockers and benzodiazepines have been used and appear to be more successful than heavy doses of tranquillisers.

Dr Kiyo Kitahara, a Japanese law graduate, has developed a school where autistic children are regimented in a near-military manner and has achieved a high measure of success. Another method, 'holding therapy', invented by an animal behaviourist, Nico Tinbergen and his wife, and developed by a New York psychiatrist, Martha Walsh, has also had considerable success.

Autistic children need specialised educational help but with as much integration as possible into mainstream schools where the children can learn to socialise with 'normal' speaking children.

Dental care

Autistic children should not be kept waiting and sessions should be brief. Eye to eye contact is often difficult to achieve, however autistic people seem to have a high degree of peripheral vision. Constant repetition of procedures is necessary so that the patient accepts a routine.

In some instances cariogenic foods are given as rewards in behaviour modification techniques and parents and carers should be encouraged to use dentally acceptable alternatives.

Admission to hospital for treatment as an inpatient should be avoided if at all possible as this involves a sudden change of situation which may be very disturbing for the autistic person.

Dementia

Dementia is described as a progressive interrelated deterioration caused by disease or injury to the brain. It is a symptom rather than a diagnosis and the aetiology should be sought in case a reversible cause exists. Such reversible causes include cerebral tumours, subdural haematoma, hypothyroidism, vitamin B_{12} deficiency and low pressure hydrocephalus. Regrettably, most patients with dementia have no such treatable cause but rather a form of cerebral atrophy often due to multiple small cerebral infarcts. Rarer causes include Creutzfeldt-Jakob disease (due to a slow virus), Huntington's disease or chronic progressive traumatic encephalopathy (this may develop in boxers as a result of repeated head injuries, even after they have ceased to box).

There is a gradual fall in mental performance; this is obviously relative, in that a patient with an IQ of 150 that falls to 120, is nevertheless suffering from dementia even though 120 is still a high level.

Alzheimer's disease

Alzheimer's disease was named after a German neurologist Alois Alzheimer who in 1907 described the microscopic changes that occurred in the brain.

Alzheimer's disease is the most common form of pre-senile or senile dementia. There is a progressive impairment in the ability to learn, to remember, and to think and the capacity to reason gradually deteriorates. In the UK nearly 10% of the population over the age of 65 and more than 20% over the age of 80 years progressively deteriorate in their intellect, memory and personality. It is estimated that about half of these people have Alzheimer's disease.

Although the cause is unknown, there appears to be an abnormality related to chromosome 21. This may explain the relationship between Down's syndrome and Alzheimer's disease, those with Down's syndrome develop dementia at a much earlier age than the average for the 'normal' population.

Alzheimer's disease is not thought to be an inherited disease; however, there may be a predisposition to the condition in some families. Investigations have shown that there is a higher level of aluminium in the brains of Alzheimer's sufferers than there is in the normal brain. A form of dementia may occur in patients on haemodialysis if exposed to dialysis fluid high in aluminium. This type of dementia responds to the drug desferrioxamine injected regularly intravenously.

The start of dementia is very gradual and it may be difficult to diagnose. Memory loss, inability to grasp new ideas and repetitiveness may be confused with the normal ageing process. When the condition is more advanced, there may be confusion regarding the time of day, forgetfulness of names of family and friends, gas left unlit, wandering around the streets at night and wearing inappropriate clothes. The progress of the disease is uncertain and varies considerably from one individual to another. Memory loss may become a major problem and there may be a loss of the normal routines regarding everyday life.

Those with the condition are probably unaware that they are dementing. Sadly, the effects are all too apparent to the carers.

Medical management

The effect of Alzheimer's disease on the partner and family is disastrous. When the dementia is severe, the patient and their family require much help and supervision and ultimately institutionalised care may be necessary.

Dental care

This depends on the patient's acceptance and co-operation. It is important to maintain the quality of life, but this changes as the condition advances. As the patient becomes more dependent on the carer for feeding and oral hygiene, prevention of infection and the removal of pain become more important than mastication and appearance. A survey of members of the Alzheimer's Disease Society showed that carers attached great importance to the provision of dental care for their relatives. It is important to ensure that the teeth are conserved before the dementia becomes too advanced as in the later stages of the disease dental treatment may be impossible.

Huntington's chorea

Huntington's chorea is an inherited degenerative condition of the central nervous system resulting in involuntary movements and mental dementia. 'Chorea' comes from the Greek word meaning 'to dance' and describes the involuntary movements. Although the condition had previously been recognised, the first person to produce a detailed account was Dr George Huntington, an American, in 1872.

The average age of onset is usually between 35 and 40 years and the illness runs a course of about 15 years. It affects both sexes and is transmitted by an autosomal dominant gene (**16**) which means that there is a 50:50 chance of inheriting the condition. As the symptoms frequently do not become apparent until mid-life, decisions may have to be made in ignorance about marriage and having a family. As yet it is not possible to reliably predict whether an individual has inherited the condition, although there are tests available which may give a reasonable degree of accuracy.

The early symptoms are slight, uncontrollable muscular movements that gradually increase in severity. Co-ordination becomes difficult and there is excessive weight loss as the patient may require around 5,000 calories a day. There may be difficulty in swallowing and in speech.

As the person loses control of their movements bowls with plate guards may prevent food from being pushed off the plate. A non-slip mat also helps to maintain the person's independence. A double handled cup with a spout may help in drinking, and knives and forks with large handles make feeding easier (**77**).

As the disease progresses, the person may no longer be able to feed themselves and chewing may be impossible.

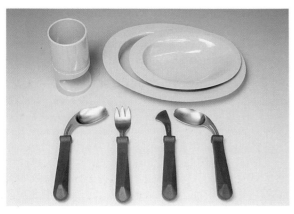

77 Plates with guards and cutlery with enlarged handles which are easier to grip.

Medical management

There is no effective therapy although haloperidol or tetrabenazine may suppress movements. Side effects include drowsiness and depression. Support is needed for the family and sooner or later institutionalised care is necessary.

Dental care

Patients with Huntington's chorea have a high energy consumption and therefore require frequent meals which tend to be high in carbohydrate and cariogenic. They also have difficulty in manipulating a toothbrush. The wearing of dentures may prove impossible in the later stages of the disease, therefore good oral hygiene measures by the patient and their carer are essential and the restriction of food intake to 4 times a day is beneficial.

Cerebrovascular Disease

Cerebrovascular disease is the commonest neurological condition in the Western world. Cerebrovascular disease is due to cerebral arteriosclerosis and the risk factors are similar to those of ischaemic heart disease, notably hypercholesterolaemia, hypertension, smoking and diabetes.

Cerebrovascular disease may be classified according to the nature and severity of the cerebral insult.

Transient ischaemic attacks

A transient ischaemic attack (TIA) is a temporary neurological deficit lasting for less than 24 hours. It may, however, presage the development of more serious and permanent neurological damage. Such a TIA is usually secondary to emboli, either from an atherosclerotic plaque in the aorta, the carotid artery and its branches, or from the heart itself.

Cerebral infarction

Cerebral infarction is due to either an embolism that fails to dissolve thus producing occlusion of a cerebral vessel, or thrombosis of an artery resulting in the loss of function of that portion of the brain which it supplies. Such infarctions produce the clinical features of a 'stroke'.

The most commonly involved vessel in cerebral infarction is the middle cerebral artery. Occlusion of the proximal part of the artery results in contralateral hemiplegia and hemisensory loss. If the dominant hemisphere is involved aphasia (loss of speech) results.

Lesser neurological deficits may occur if more distal portions of this artery are occluded and dysphasia (difficulty in speaking) occurs.

The clinical diagnosis of cerebral infarction may be confirmed by computerised tomography, but the clinical findings are very characteristic. The prognosis is unpredictable: about 35% die in hospital, particularly the elderly.

Medical management

Full supportive care is required in the initial stages, with fluid replacement by appropriate means, reassurance, physiotherapy, and occupational and speech therapy. Anticoagulants may be prescribed if an embolus is considered to be the cause.

The extent of recovery depends on the site and size of the infarction. Although maximal recovery occurs in the first few weeks after a stroke, it must be remembered that some recovery may occur up to one year after the initial ictus.

Dental care

This should be avoided in the initial stages after a stroke, as the prognosis is uncertain.

Oral hygiene is, however, of paramount importance, particularly if the patient is unable to swallow. Moreover, the patient inadvertently tends to accumulate food and, therefore, plaque in the mouth on the same side as the hemiplegia.

When the patient is neurologically stable, dental treatment may be undertaken but general anaesthesia should be avoided for 6 months after a stroke. It should be remembered that although an aphasic or dysphasic patient may be unable to communicate verbally, comprehension may not be affected and all procedures should be carefully explained.

Cerebral haemorrhage

This may be classified according to the origin and site, either intracranial or subarachnoid haemorrhage. In intracranial haemorrhage there is rupture of an arteriosclerotic vessel that has been long exposed to hypertension or made ischaemic by a local thrombus. Occasionally there may be rupture of a congenital aneurysm of the circle of Willis.

The clinical picture bears many similarities to that of cerebral infarction, indeed it may be difficult to distinguish between them without computerised tomography, although a sudden onset of neurological symptoms, increasing in severity, associated with a severe headache is characteristic.

Medical management and dental care

Similar to the treatment for cerebral infarction.

Subarachnoid haemorrhage

This occurs as a result of haemorrhage into the subarachnoid space, usually due to the rupture of a congenital intracranial aneurysm.

There is a sudden onset of a severe headache. As blood is very irritant to the meninges, vomiting may occur, as well as stiffness of the neck, drowsiness and coma. The diagnosis may be made by a lumbar puncture or computerised tomography.

A total of 35% of patients succumb from the initial haemorrhage and a further 15% die from subsequent haemorrhages in the next few weeks. It is therefore necessary in young patients to identify any potential aneurysms as surgical obliteration may be possible to prevent re-bleeding.

Medical management

Initially, bed rest is recommended. When the patient is neurologically stable, angiography may be undertaken and, if appropriate, surgery.

Dental care

Similar care as for patients with cerebral infarction.

10 Neuromuscular Disorders

Muscular Dystrophy

Muscular dystrophy is an inherited condition affecting skeletal muscles and is progressive and degenerative. The most common form of muscular dystrophy is the Duchenne or childhood form. The incidence is about 0.14 per 1000 children and classically occurs only in boys. It is caused by an X-linked recessive gene (**14**) occurring in about 1 in 20 of the general population and is transmitted by a female carrier. Affected boys appear to be normal during the first year of life but may be late in sitting up and may not walk until 18 months of age or even later. Difficulty in climbing stairs may be an early symptom of the condition. The disease progresses fairly rapidly and by the end of the first decade they may be seriously disabled and confined to a wheelchair. By the end of the second decade there is susceptibility to pulmonary infections and involvement of the cardiac muscles resulting in death.

About 25% of affected individuals have some degree of learning difficulty. However most boys are usually only too well aware of the outcome of their condition. Survival into the late twenties is rare.

Medical management

Tragically, there is no effective treatment and there is a gradual deterioration. Supportive treatment for the patients and their families is essential.

Genetic counselling is important, as about one-third of the cases occur in families with other boys with the condition.

Dental care

Regular visits are necessary to maintain oral health, as in the later stages there may be limited opening of the mouth, due to muscular contractions making any form of dental treatment extremely difficult. General anaesthetics must be avoided as there is poor chest movement and there is an added risk of cardiac arrest and malignant hyperpyrexia.

Myasthenia Gravis

Myasthenia gravis is a neuromuscular disorder characterised by muscular weakness due to a defect in neuromuscular transmission.

The nerve impulse to a muscle involves the release of acetylcholine at the nerve endings. Myasthenia gravis appears to be an autoimmune disease in which the acetylcholine receptors on the surface of the skeletal muscle fibres become coated with acetylcholine receptor antibodies, thus impairing neuromuscular transmission.

There is a high incidence of enlargement of the thymus or thymoma. The incidence of myasthenia gravis is 1 in 20,000 and is more common in females on a 3:2 basis.

The muscles often affected are the ocular (producing proptosis or diplopia), facial, laryngeal, pharyngeal and respiratory. There is progressive weakness of the muscles when in use, with rapid recovery after a period of rest. Symptoms typically occur in the evening and disappear after a night's rest.

Medical management

The first line of treatment is with anticholinesterases which enhance neuromuscular transmission in the voluntary and involuntary muscles. If this is not successful, corticosteroids may be given in conjunction with the anticholinesterases. Plasmapheresis prior to thymectomy may cure 30–45% of patients.

Dental care

General anaesthesia should be avoided because of the weakness of the respiratory muscles. There may be excessive salivation as a side effect of the anti-cholinesterase drugs. Patients are more comfortable when treated in the upright position.

Infection or stress may cause a myasthenic crisis during which the patient may have difficulty in clearing secretions from the throat and develop respiratory distress which may be life threatening.

Guillain–Barré Syndrome

There are several synonyms for this syndrome, including Landry-Guillain–Barré syndrome. The first description of a type of ascending paralysis was published by Landry in French in 1859. The classical publication detailing the symptoms appeared in a Parisian medical bulletin by Landry, Guillain, Barré and Strohl in 1915.

This acute or subacute condition affects the nerve roots and peripheral nerves in a diffuse manner, resulting in weakness, loss of sensation, pain and possible paralysis. It occurs sporadically and affects people of all ages and both sexes. It usually follows a viral or bacterial infection but has also been associated with leukaemia, lymphoma and post-immunisation. Its aetiology is unknown but an autoimmune mechanism has been suggested.

Clinically, there is a general weakness of the lower limbs with paraesthesia that spreads to involve the arms and the respiratory muscles. There may also be cranial involvement, with unilateral or bilateral facial palsy.

Medical management

Respiratory paralysis severe enough to necessitate mechanical ventilation occurs in 10–25% of patients.

However the prognosis is good, as the condition usually improves spontaneously, although there may be some residual weakness and recovery may take up to 2 years.

Dental care

There may be a risk with general anaesthesia if the respiratory muscles are affected, and dental treatment should be postponed until recovery has occurred.

11 Musculoskeletal Disorders

The term 'arthritis' is used to describe an inflammatory condition of the joint. Joint inflammation may be caused by infection, trauma, degenerative joint disease, endocrine disorders, or it may be idiopathic.

Juvenile Chronic Arthritis

Juvenile chronic arthritis is defined as an inflammatory arthritis occurring before the age of 16 years and now embraces Still's disease, first described by Sir George Frederick Still in 1896, the first professor of paediatrics in the UK. It is a very variable condition and there are several clinical subgroups.

The aetiology is not known. It may be the result of infection or it may be due to an autoimmune reaction. It is characterised by fever, skin rash, lymphadenopathy and inflammatory arthritis, usually affecting four or more joints. There is a chronic non-suppurative inflammation of the synovium. The joints become swollen, warm, and tender to touch and painful to move.

Many children eventually develop adult forms of polyarthritis, such as rheumatoid arthritis, ankylosing spondylitis and various forms of connective tissue diseases, the commonest being systemic lupus erythematosus.

Medical management

This is aimed at preserving the function of the joints. First line therapy consists of anti-inflammatory drugs, usually the non-steroidal anti-inflammatory drugs (NSAIDs) such as acetylsalicylic acid (aspirin). There are however a number of second line drugs, used when the NSAIDs are inadequate or ineffective, including sulphasalazine and immunosuppressive therapy with steroids and azathioprine. Corticosteroids may result in retardation of growth if used for prolonged periods, alternate day steroids may result in fewer side effects and in particular less growth retardation in children.

Intra-articular corticosteroids may be used.

Eyes should be checked regularly by an ophthalmologist to detect iridocyclitis and thus treat it at an early stage with corticosteroid drops in order to prevent blindness.

Daily exercises, such as swimming, should be encouraged, and also the wearing of supporting splints in order to prevent joint deformities. Rest splints are frequently used at night to support joints in their optimum position.

Dental care

Oral hygiene measures are extremely important as many children take drugs in syrup form (see page 114). There may be involvement of the temperomandibular joint resulting in restricted opening. General anaesthesia may present problems due to limitation in the movement of the chest. Transient bacteraemia is unlikely to cause problems, but oral sepsis should be prevented.

Rheumatoid Arthritis

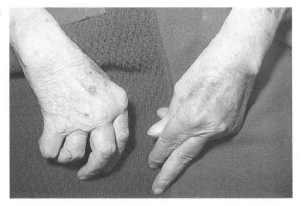

78 Distortion of the hands as a result of rheumatoid arthritis.

This is the most common chronic inflammatory disease of joints, affecting about 3% of the population and occurring more frequently in women. Although it may occur at any age there is a peak in women aged 35–55 years. Initially the small joints of the hands and wrists are particularly affected (**78**) and this may be associated with systemic manifestations, including weight loss, lethargy and depression. Gradually, more joints are affected, accompanied by morning stiffness which may take several hours before easing. The joints are swollen and tender.

Men are usually affected at 40–60 years of age. The onset may be acute with tenderness and pain in a number of joints, or it may be more insidious. There may also be subcutaneous rheumatoid nodules.

Medical management

Bed rest is advisable during the acute phase of the disease. Non-steroidal anti-inflammatory drugs, such as acetylsalicylic acid (aspirin) are effective in many patients. Other drugs available if aspirin is not effective include gold compounds, antimalarials, penicillamine, sulphasalazine, steroids (either intra-articular or oral) and immunosuppressants. These drugs are not without their side effects, which include anaemia and platelet abnormalities.

After the control of inflammation, exercise is essential to maintain movement in the joints and strengthen the muscles. Splinting and other orthopaedic measures may be necessary to prevent contracture of the joints. Various aids are available to help maintain independence.

Dental care

The main cause for concern regarding dental treatment is when there is possible involvement of the cervical spine, producing gross instability of the atlanto-occipital joint which, if the neck is flexed, may result in compression of the spinal cord and spasticity. Patients should have X-rays of the cervical spine to identify those at risk.

Drugs may give rise to potential problems – bleeding tendencies secondary to NSAIDs, suppression of the bone marrow as a result of gold salts or penicillamine, and adrenal suppression as a result of steroids.

Good oral hygiene can be difficult to maintain. The handles of toothbrushes may require modification so they can be held more easily (**70**). Temporomandibular joint surgery may be necessary if there is severe involvement of the joint. There may be difficulty with access if the patient is in a wheelchair. Stiffness is worse in the morning, so dental appointments may be better in the afternoon.

Osteogenesis Imperfecta

Osteogenesis imperfecta (fragilitas ossium) is a disorder of the mesenchyme and its derivatives resulting in the abnormal synthesis of collagen, affecting mainly that of the bone. The cortical bone is much thinner than normal and the bones are fragile, leading to frequent fractures with minimal trauma (pathological fractures). It is of autosomal dominant inheritance (**16**) with an incidence of about 1:30,000 live births (**79**).

Following fractures, callus forms which is then replaced by weakened bone. There are deformities of the limbs mainly as a result of the fractures, and there is excessive laxity of the ligaments resulting in hypermobility of the joints.

The sclera, which is derived from mesenchyme, is thin and this allows the pigmented choroid to shine through giving a bluish hue (**80**). Dentinogenesis imperfecta (opalescent dentine) may be associated with osteogenesis imperfecta but both canoccur independently (**81**).

There are various forms of the condition. In the congenital form (Type II) fractures may occur in utero and the baby is born with deformities and about 50% are stillborn. Fractures may also occur during delivery and most affected babies die soon after birth.

In the tarda form (Type I) the baby appears normal at birth and fractures do not usually occur until the end of the first year. The incidence of fractures reduces dramatically at puberty. Those who are severely affected may be confined to a wheelchair.

Medical management

Prevention of fractures is not easy and parents must guard against being overprotective. Every fracture must be carefully treated in order to prevent the bones healing with a deformity.

Dental care

Care must be taken during extractions to avoid fracturing the mandible. To avoid applying pressure, it may be necessary to reflect a flap and remove supporting bone.

Dislocation of the temperomandibular joint may occur during dental treatment as a result of the lax ligaments. Although the dislocation can be reduced, the condyle may fracture in the process. Props and gags should be used with extreme care under general anaesthesia.

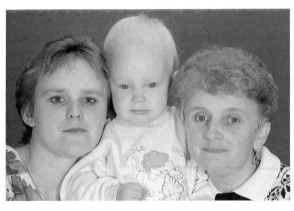

79 A 2¹/₂-year-old girl with her mother and maternal grandmother, all affected by osteogenesis imperfecta with associated dentinogenesis imperfecta.

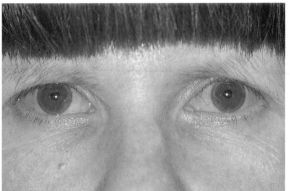

80 Blue sclera in patient with osteogenesis imperfecta.

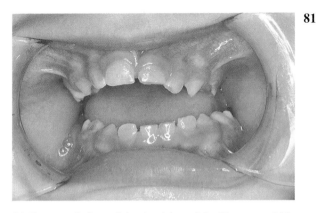

81 Intra-oral view of the dentition of the 2¹/₂-year-old in **79**.

Dentinogenesis imperfecta (hereditary opalescent dentine)

This condition is also inherited as an autosomal dominant gene. The teeth appear opalescent due to the discoloured dentine shining through the enamel (**82**). The crowns are bulbous with short roots. The dentine is poorly formed and gives insufficient support for the enamel. Enamel fractures off and there is rapid attrition of the dentine (**83**). There is sclerosis and calcification of the pulp chamber at an early age and the remaining pulpal tissue has a poor blood supply and becomes non-vital. This may cause no problems but, following a bacteraemia, infection may occur in the apical region (**84**).

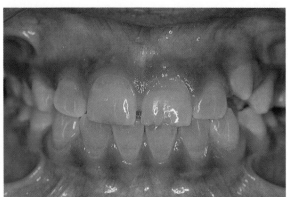

82 Opalescent appearance of the permanent dentition in a patient with dentinogenesis imperfecta.

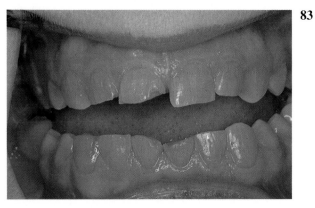

83 Permanent dentition in a 16-year-old with dentinogenesis imperfecta showing excessive attrition and chipping of the incisal edges.

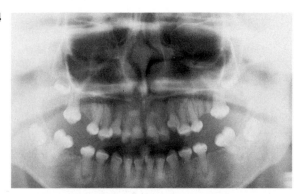

84 Orthopantomogram of a patient with dentinogenesis imperfecta. Note the bulbous crowns and short roots. The first permanent molars have all had to be extracted due to apical infection in spite of the fact that she had a caries-free dentition.

Dental care

This depends on the severity of the condition. In mild cases composite restorations or crowns may be possible. In the more severe cases mouthguards should be constructed for the patient to wear at night to prevent attrition.

Although it may be possible to crown the teeth it is distressing for patients to lose them ultimately as a result of apical infection. As a result of sclerosis and calcification of the pulp chambers endodontic treatment is not usually feasible in the posterior teeth; in the anterior teeth it may be possible to apicect the teeth and place retrograde root fillings.

It is advisable to retain the teeth for as long as possible. As a result of attrition the construction of overdentures may be necessary to maintain the vertical dimension and improve the lower facial height, thus improving the facial contour (**85–88**).

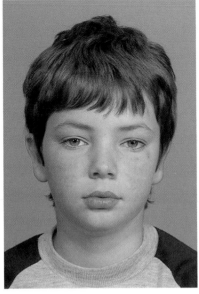

85 A 10-year-old boy with dentinogenesis imperfecta. There is reduction in the lower facial height due to attrition of his permanent dentition

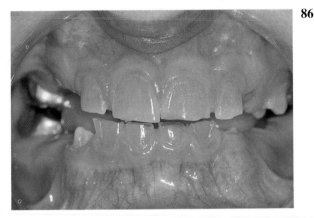

86 Intra-oral view of the boy in **85**.

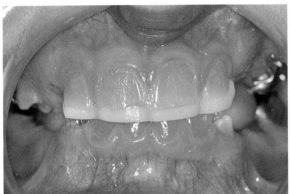

87 Appliance to open the bite anteriorly (same patient as **85**).

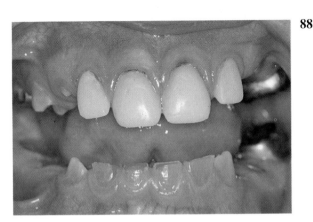

88 Composite restorations have been placed on the permanent anterior incisor teeth as an interim measure (same patient as **85**).

12 Dermatological Disorders

Scleroderma

Scleroderma is a rare progressive disease of unknown aetiology. It affects tissue of mesenchymal origin in which it causes degenerative changes and hypertrophy of the collagenous component of the skin and subcutaneous tissues. It occurs in a progressive systemic form and a localised form. The disease is insidious in onset; there may be prodromal symptoms of pain and swelling of the joints and the affected skin shows inflammatory changes. If the oesophagus is affected there may be difficulty in swallowing. Other organs may also be involved, including the bowel, lung, heart and kidney.

Morphoea is the linear or more localised form of the condition. It is benign and self limiting. During the acute phase there is inflammation, followed by fibrosis and scarring and contractures.

The skin adheres to the subcutaneous tissue and appears smooth and waxy (**89**). In children, growth may be affected as a result of ischaemia to the area, pressure and lack of mobility (**90**). Occasionally there is an indurated band affecting the scalp or forehead giving rise to scleroderma en coup de sabre. The mouth may be reduced in size (**91**) and alveolar growth affected (**92**). The teeth in the affected area are firm in spite of a widening of the periodontal membrane. The disease runs a chronic course.

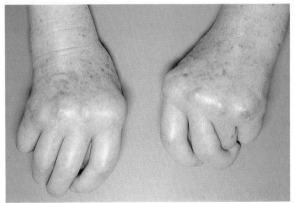

89 The deformed, smooth and waxy appearance of the hands of a patient with generalised scleroderma (courtesy of Mr J. Hamburger).

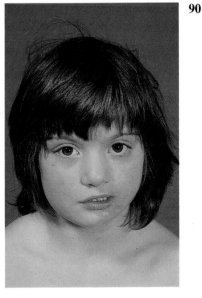

90 Scleroderma affecting the left side of the face resulting in facial hemiatrophy (courtesy of Professor T.D. Foster).

91

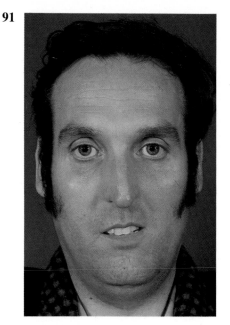

92

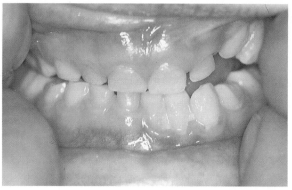

92 Oral view of the girl in **90**. There is gingival recession and loss of alveolar bone on the left side in the mouth (courtesy of Professor T.D. Foster and Churchill Livingstone).

91 Generalised scleroderma. The skin is adherent to the underlying tissues and the mouth is reduced in size.

Medical management

The prognosis is poor for the generalised form. Treatment is to provide symptomatic relief. Corticosteroids may be helpful for those with disabling myositis. Treatment for associated hypertension is necessary and chronic renal replacement therapy may be required if renal failure occurs. There is no drug that affects the course of the disease. Appropriate treatment of reflux oesophagitis and oesophageal strictures may be indicated.

Dental care

Preventive treatment is of the utmost importance in order to avoid extractions in an affected area. Access to the mouth may, however, be difficult because of the fibrosis of the skin.

Oesophagitis or oesophageal reflux may cause erosion of the teeth (*see* page 115).

Epidermolysis Bullosa

Epidermolysis bullosa is the name given to a number of genetically determined skin conditions in which the skin and mucous membrane blister as a result of mechanical trauma. The condition, though rare, occurs world-wide.

A number of distinct types have been described and may be grouped into three main categories: epidermolysis bullosa simplex, epidermolysis bullosa dystrophica and junctional epidermolysis bullosa.

Epidermolysis bullosa simplex

This non-scarring form is autosomal dominant (**16**). Blisters are usually present at birth and are often confined to the hands and feet. Although the condition is not very severe, some people have difficulty walking and others find working with their hands difficult.

Epidermolysis bullosa dystrophica

The disease is inherited as an autosomal dominant or autosomal recessive trait and appears to be most severe when inherited in the recessive form. Dystrophica means mutilating and in this form of the condition there is a tendency to healing of the blisters with atrophic scarring resulting in considerable disfigurement (**93–95**). Bullae form readily when the mucosa is touched and the resultant scarring particularly of the lips may lead to contracture and further difficulties with access. Blisters in the oesophagus may result in stricture, making swallowing difficult and food may have to be liquidised. There may also be scarring of the buccal mucosa which can affect eating and talking. Fusion of the fingers and loss of the nails result in severe deformities. Intelligence is not affected, indeed many with the condition are of above average intelligence which makes it even more difficult for them to accept the limitations imposed by the condition.

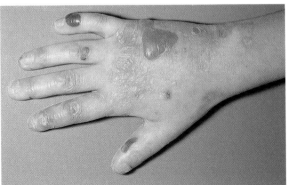

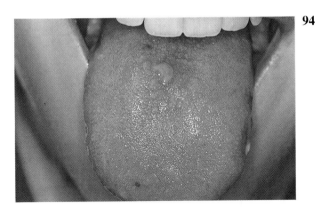

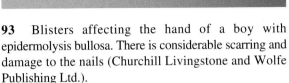

93　Blisters affecting the hand of a boy with epidermolysis bullosa. There is considerable scarring and damage to the nails (Churchill Livingstone and Wolfe Publishing Ltd.).

94　Intra-oral view of the boy in **93**, showing a blister on the dorsum of the tongue.

95　Permanent dentition of the boy in **93**, showing evidence of periodontal breakdown in the lower incisor region in spite of quite good oral hygiene.

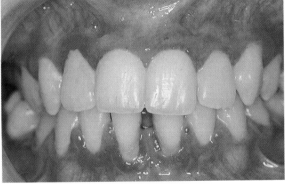

Junctional epidermolysis bullosa

Although this is a non-scarring form, it is likely to result in death in infancy or early childhood. It is an autosomal recessive condition. There are usually large blisters present at birth and septicaemia is a frequent cause of death.

Medical management

Skin care is directed at prevention of trauma wherever possible and providing optimal conditions for the healing of the blisters and ulcers.

Dental care

Preventive advice regarding a non-cariogenic diet is essential. Advice should be given on the use of a soft toothbrush to maintain oral hygiene and chlorhexidine mouthwashes to prevent the accumulation of plaque. Cleansing with sponges or cotton wool buds may also be beneficial.

Regular dental examinations are essential in order to detect and treat early lesions and thereby avoid extractions. Retention of the teeth is of the utmost importance as these patients will be unable to tolerate dentures.

Great care must be taken in order to avoid cotton wool rolls becoming stuck to the mucosa and saliva ejectors damaging or traumatising the mucosa.

If a general anaesthetic is required care must be taken during intubation and lifting and moving the patient. All those involved should be aware of the vulnerability of the skin.

Ectodermal Dysplasia

96 A 7-year-old boy with ecto-dermal dysplasia. There is evidence of frontal bossing, rather prominent ears and fine, sparse hair.

Ectodermal dysplasia is a disorder affecting the tissues derived from the ectoderm. This condition occurs in two main forms (Clouston types) — anhidrotic and hidrotic.

The hidrotic is the more common form and has an autosomal dominant inheritance. The anhidrotic form is X-linked recessive, occurring in its full expression only in males. In both forms there may be frontal bossing, depressed nasal bridge, protruberant and everted lips and rather prominent ears. The hair is very fine and sparse and is usually blond. Eyebrows and eyelashes are often missing and there may be pigmentation around the eyes (**96**).

In the anhidrotic form, in addition, there is a reduction in the number of sebaceous glands and sweat glands, which results in a dry skin and an intolerance to heat. The palms of the hands show absence or reduction of sweat pores. There is difficulty in maintaining body temperature as cooling cannot occur on the surface of the skin by sensible or insensible perspiration. Infections may lead to death in infancy as a result of hypothermia. There may be a link with cot deaths.

There may also be a reduction in salivary flow and lacrimal flow and it may be necessary to use eye and nose drops several times a day in order to prevent damage to the cornea.

There is usually an associated reduction in the number of teeth (hypodontia) (**97**). Rarely is there total absence of teeth (anodontia). The teeth which are present are more parallel-sided or even conical in form (**98**). As a result of failure of development of the dentition there is a reduction in the lower facial height.

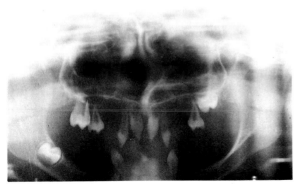

97 Orthopantomogram of the boy in **96** who has hypodontia with few permanent teeth.

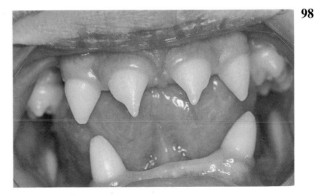

98 Intra-oral view of boy in **96** following the eruption of the upper permanent central incisors which are very conical in form. The other teeth present are the primary canines.

Medical management

In the anhidrotic type this involves maintenance of body temperature by keeping the body cool either by tepid showers or baths, wearing a damp T-shirt if over heated, and using air conditioning or fans in the bedroom.

Dental care

Prevention of dental disease is of the utmost importance in order to maintain the teeth that are present for as long as possible, particularly when there are no permanent successors. A multi-disciplinary approach is often required which may involve orthodontic and advanced restorative techniques (**99**). In those people with severe hypodontia it is likely that prosthetic treatment, possibly involving the restoration of facial height with over-dentures may be required (**100–102**).

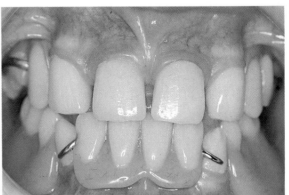

99 Porcelain crowns bonded to the upper primary canines and permanent central incisors. The only preparation of the teeth was removal of the pointed tips. The missing lower teeth were restored with a skeleton metal denture (same patient as **96**).

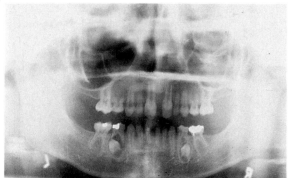

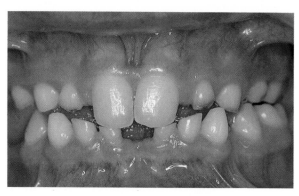

100 Orthopantomogram of an 8-year-old girl with marked hypodontia.

101 Intra-oral view of the girl in **100** who has lack of alveolar growth due to failure of development of many permanent teeth; in the maxillary arch only the central incisors and first permanent molars have formed.

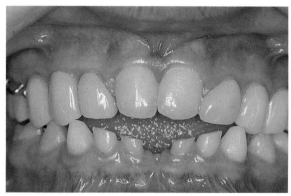

102 Over-denture to improve the appearance and restore the occlusal height. Subsequently, treatment will be required in the lower arch (same patient as **100**).

13 Sensory Disturbances

Hearing Impairment

Hearing is the principal sensory pathway through which speech and verbal communication develop. Even mild impairments of hearing may prevent the normal development of a child. Impaired hearing may not be obvious and the child may be thought to have learning difficulties. As a result of impaired hearing, speech development may be poor and affected children may be difficult to understand. Stimulation from parents, peer groups, teachers and the world at large is very important in the development of the child. If this input is lacking then those who are deaf grow up further disadvantaged.

The three main types of hearing loss are discussed below.

Conductive

Conductive hearing loss is due to interference of sound through the outer and middle ear. There are many causes, both congenital and acquired. There may be congenital abnormalities of the external ear, the ossicles, canal or ear drum, as occurs in some cranio-facial abnormalities (**103,104**), or there may be acquired problems, such as wax in the outer ear or fluid in the middle ear, both of which may prevent the transmission of sound to the middle ear.

103,104 Front and side view of boy with a first arch defect. He has a vestigial pinna and abnormalities of the middle and inner ear with loss of hearing on that side.

103

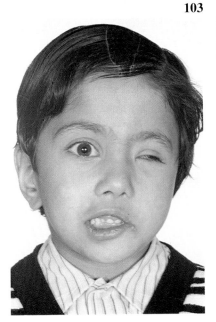

104

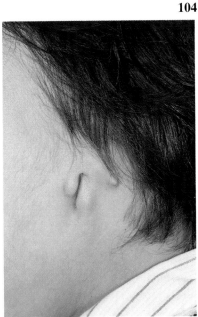

Medical management

Conductive hearing loss may be managed by medical or surgical means.

Sensorineural

Sensorineural hearing loss is due to a defect of the auditory nerve or the cochlea hair cells. This may be caused by viral infections (particularly mumps and intrauterine rubella), certain drugs (streptomycin group, aminoglycosides, high doses of diuretics and some anti-cancer drugs), vascular occlusion, loud noises in industry and loud music

Medical management

The condition is usually irreversible and does not respond to medical or surgical intervention. However, there have been advances in recent years with cochlear implants. These patients may also suffer from an annoying and disturbing ringing in the ears (tinnitus), vestibular problems and vertigo.

Central auditory defects

In this condition there is interference with the transmission of sound through the central auditory brain stem and cortical pathways. This may be due to pre-, peri-, or post-natal factors. This form of hearing loss may also occur in old age.

Dental care

The main difficulty experienced is that of communication. These people are not mentally handicapped; they have normal intelligence and are just deaf.

In young children, sign language may be necessary. Older children and adults may have learnt to lip read. It is therefore essential that the patient can see the speaker's face so that he or she can see the expression and lip movements. Lip movements need to be clear but not exaggerated. The wearing of a mask makes it very difficult for the patient to understand.

Simple advice from the Royal National Institute for the Deaf: a deaf person is most likely to understand when the speaker talks in a clear voice, slightly slower than usual but with a normal rhythm, so that the deaf person can both hear and see the speaker.

If a hearing aid is worn the patient should be asked to switch it off before using the high speed turbine or air scaler.

Visual Impairment

There is a wide range of visual loss, from those who are able to define shapes and light and darkness to those unable to perceive light at all.

Cataracts

Cataracts are due to denaturation of the lens. Congenital cataracts occur as a result of rubella infection of the fetus during the first trimester. This used to be quite common, but has become much less so in Western countries in recent years due to immunisation programmes (*see* page 105). The most common cause of cataracts is ageing, when there is gradual loss of vision. Steroid therapy may also be involved in the aetiology of some cataracts

Cataracts also occur in diabetic people causing blindness. A further major cause of loss of vision in diabetics is retinopathy, which particularly affects insulin-dependant diabetics (IDDM) (*see* pages 51–53). This may be delayed if the diabetic state and blood pressure are well controlled and smoking is avoided. It is important that diabetic people should have annual checks with an opthalmologist for retinopathy.

Medical management

Vision may be maintained in the early stages of cataract development by change of spectacle prescriptions. When there has been loss of useful vision, removal of the lens may be necessary with replacement by a prosthetic lens, contact lenses or corrective spectacles.

Trauma

Trauma, particularly in young people, may result in penetration of the eye and loss of sight. Other causes of blindness are glaucoma and retinitis pigmentosa.

Medical management

Children who are blind or partially sighted require education in special schools, many of which are residential.

Dental care

The patient should be encouraged to feel the chair and equipment and full explanations should be given. Physical contact is of the utmost importance. Sudden unexplained movements should be avoided.

14 Infections

Rubella (German Measles)

Rubella is a contagious disease caused by an RNA virus spread by close contact or aerosols. It is usually a mild condition in children, comprising a rash, fever and enlarged and tender lymph nodes in the head and neck region. The condition may be more serious in older children and adults.

If an expectant mother contracts rubella the virus can cross the placenta and infect the fetus. This may result in an abortion or a baby with rubella syndrome. The effects are most severe if the mother develops rubella during the first 4 months of pregnancy, but problems may also occur if the mother has had rubella 3 months prior to conception.

The classical triad of deafness, cardiac defects and eye defects. which occur in the rubella syndrome, was first described by Sir Norman Gregg in 1941. In about 40% of cases there is also mental retardation. There is a high incidence of premature babies and low birth weight babies.

Medical management

If the mother contracts rubella during the first few months of pregnancy, a therapeutic abortion should be considered in view of the potential effects on the fetus. It is hoped, however, with active prevention of rubella by immunisation, that the incidence of the rubella syndrome will decrease dramatically. Immunisation is recommended along with mumps and measles at about 15 months of age. All teenage girls should receive the vaccine if not already protected.

Dental care

There may be missing teeth and abnormalities in the shape of the teeth, particularly the primary molars.

If there is cardiac involvement, prophylactic antibiotics are necessary for invasive dental treatment. General anaesthesia may be necessary if co-operation is impossible due to a lack of understanding.

Encephalitis

The commonest cause of encephalitis in the UK is secondary to a viral infection for which mumps, measles, echo and coxsackie viruses may be responsible. Less commonly, herpes simplex and zoster and the Epstein–Barr virus (glandular fever) may be the cause.

The two main features of encephalitis are headache and alteration in the state of consciousness, which may vary from lethargy and drowsiness to stupor and coma. The onset may be sudden or insidious and recovery may be equally variable depending on the aetiological agent.

Diagnosis is made by a combination of clinical features and the examination of the cerebrospinal fluid (CSF). It may be necessary to carry out an encephalogram and a CT scan to exclude a focal lesion.

Medical management

There is no specific treatment unless caused by herpes when acyclovir has been found to produce a dramatic improvement.

Dental care

This should be delayed until the outcome of the encephalitis is confirmed.

Meningitis

Meningitis is an inflammation of the meninges of the brain and spinal cord. It may be due to bacteria, viruses or fungal infections.

There is a fever, headache, vomiting and a stiff neck. Convulsions may occur in young children. It is impor-tant that a precise diagnosis is obtained by examination of the CSF. The patient may be severely ill but recovery can be complete. However, in young children there may be permanent cerebral damage resulting in learning difficulties, deafness and hydrocephalus.

Medical management

As a result of examination of the CSF, the appropriate antibiotics must be given as soon as possible.

Dental care

Treatment should not present any problems following recovery unless there has been permanent brain damage when mental impairment may prevent co-operation.

Human Immunodeficiency Virus

Acquired immune deficiency syndrome (AIDS) was first described in the UK in 1981. The discovery of the virus which causes AIDS was made in France in 1983 by cultivating the cells of an infected patient and was called lymphadenopathy-associated virus (LAV). The Americans isolated a virus which they termed human T-cell lymphocytic virus Type III (HTVL III). The term human immunodeficiency viruses or HIV is now generally accepted.

HIV is an RNA virus of the retrovirus class and is believed to have originated from the monkey. A high incidence of the virus has been identified in certain parts of the world, notably Africa where, in certain areas, 20% of the population has been said to be infected .

The virus has been detected in blood, semen, saliva, tears, vaginal secretions and the milk of nursing mothers. However, the virus is of low infectivity and there have been no instances reported of transmission by tears, saliva or air. There is no evidence of transmission by contact at work or school, or even by close personal contact, sharing household utensils and other facilities.

Individuals who are likely to become infected are homosexual males, intravenous drug abusers, recipients of contaminated blood or blood products, and heterosexual contacts of those affected with HIV.

Four different patterns of the disease have been identified:

- Initial infection, which may produce features of a mild viral illness, with fever, evanescent skin rash and lymphadenopathy.
- Carrier status, an asymptomatic phase with failure of eradication of the virus from the circulation.
- Generalised lymphadenopathy.
- Full blown disease with the development of severe infections, particularly opportunistic infections, such as pneumocystis carinii, as a result of destruction of the defences of the body against infections.

The first clinical manifestation of HIV infection is frequently in the mouth and oropharynx and includes candidiasis, aphthous ulcers, periodontitis and necrotising gingivitis. It is therefore important that the dental team is aware of these manifestations

Candidiasis (oral thrush) is not unusual in some patients (for example diabetics, those taking steroids or antibiotics, cancer patients and those with other debilitating diseases), but is most unusual in the mouth of a young person (105). Erythematous candidosis typically affects the palate or tongue. Again, angular cheilitis is not unusual in edentulous patients but very unusual in those who are dentate. In individuals with a fair standard of dental hygiene the presence of intractable and recurrent gingivitis, with ulceration and punched out dental papillae, that resembles acute necrotising ulcerative gingivitis and does not respond to treatment, should also arouse suspicions. Rashes on the face, either in the form of seborrhoeic dermatitis or molluscum contagiosum, must be viewed with suspicion, as should intra-oral warts and severe forms of aphthous ulceration.

Hairy leukoplakia has been observed with increasing frequency in homosexual men and patients with HIV or AIDS related complex (ARC). It occurs almost exclusively on the lateral border of the tongue as small whitish finger-like projections (106). It is not known to be pre-malignant. Kaposi's sarcoma is relatively rare in the general population but occurs in around a third of HIV/ARC patients. It occurs at the junction of the hard and soft palate as a red, blue or purple macule, papule or nodule (107).

Medical management

At present HIV infection is incurable. Treatment is aimed at preventing opportunistic infection and interrupting the replication of the cycle of HIV by using the drug zidovudine. Regrettably, this drug is not without toxicity, especially to the bone marrow, and produces a number of unpleasant side effects. Death is usually due to secondary infection, although it may be preceded by progressive dementia and renal failure.

Psychological support is also important as HIV usually afflicts the young, who are only too aware of the terminal nature of the disease.

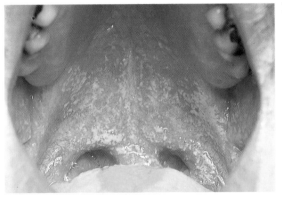

105 Candidiasis in a patient with AIDS.

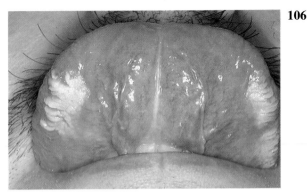

106 Hairy leucoplakia on the side of the tongue due to projections of keratinised squamous epithelium.

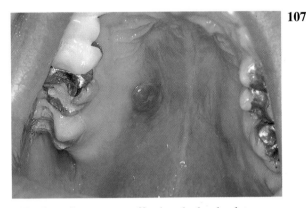

107 Kaposi's sarcoma affecting the hard palate.

Treatment should not be denied to those with HIV infection. It is estimated that the risk of acquiring HIV infection following a contaminated needle stick injury is about 0.4% in the USA. The likelihood of generating aerosols by low and high speed drills, ultrasonic scalers and irrigation or air syringes emphasises the need to wear protective eyewear, rubber gloves and a mask when working with known HIV antibody positive patients. Indeed, in view of the fact that many asymptomatic carriers remain undetected, the only safe procedure is to treat all patients in the same way.

Screening for HIV positive individuals is not permitted in the UK at the present time without the patient's consent and counselling.

Hepatitis

Hepatitis is the general term used to describe the group of inflammatory diseases which affect the liver. The cellular necrosis that results releases hepatic enzymes into the circulation and the raised level can be detected in a peripheral blood sample.

Hepatitis may be due to many causes and it is important to know the aetiology. It may be due to viral, bacterial or fungal infections, a large number of drugs including anaesthetic agents or alcohol. Of particular importance to those treating patients are the forms of hepatitis caused by viruses: hepatitis A virus, hepatitis B virus ,hepatitis C, and infectious mononucleosis (Epstein–Barr virus) are the commonest.

Hepatitis A (HAV)

This is caused by an RNA type virus, and was previously called infectious hepatitis. It is invariably transmitted by the faecal-oral route or by contamination of food or water, and the spread of infection occurs rapidly when there is poor sanitation, overcrowding and inadequate personal hygiene. Contaminated shellfish are often implicated.

Hepatitis B (HBV)

This is caused by a DNA type virus and was previously known as serum hepatitis as it is most commonly transmitted by blood or blood products. Infection may occur by direct inoculation of infected serum or plasma, by transfusion of infected blood, or through cuts and abrasions in mucosal surfaces.

Certain groups of people are particularly at risk; these include homosexual males, intravenous drug users and health care workers. Prior to the screening of blood in the UK in 1985, there was a high incidence in haemophiliacs and other recipients of blood transfusions.

HBV affects people world-wide, with a low incidence of around 5–10% in the United Kingdom and the United States, whereas in East Asia, sub-Saharan Africa and China it is as high as 80%. About 400 million people in the world are chronically infected with the hepatitis B virus, and most of them live in the developing countries. It is acquired in childhood and causes the death of parents of young children thus causing untold misery, a disease which could be avoided by immunisation.

It is impossible to make a diagnosis of the type of hepatitis from the clinical appearance, the signs and symptoms being very similar.

Many infections are sub-clinical, those who are affected more severely have flu-like symptoms, such as loss of appetite, nausea, vomiting and fever followed by jaundice. Paradoxically, the previous symptoms may regress as the jaundice worsens over a period of 1–2 weeks, and then fade over the next 2–4 weeks. The most serious consequence of HBV infection is a fulminating liver cell necrosis with a mortality of 10–15%.

Failure to eradicate the virus despite resolution of the hepatitis results in a carrier state. The frequency of carriers varies from less than 0.5% in the United Kingdom to greater than 10% in the Far East. The carrier status may be identified serologically with the presence of the surface antigen of the virus (HepBsAg). Contact with the blood or even the saliva of patients who are HepBsAg positive produces a small, but nevertheless significant, risk to the dental team.

Medical management

The spread of HAV may be prevented by rigorous personal hygiene. A vaccine has recently been developed and it is advisable for high risk groups, e.g. healthcare workers, and those travelling to, or living in, medium or high risk areas to receive immunisation.

In HBV the development of asymptomatic carriers is a cause for concern. As many as 25% of carriers can develop chronic active hepatitis with progressive liver damage and cirrhosis. The medical history may fail to reveal carriers, therefore it is essential to practice a strict protocol in all patients to prevent cross infection.

Thus, treatment should be aimed at prevention. A vaccine for Hepatitis B has been available since 1982. As yet it is too expensive for mass inoculations but it is strongly recommended that those at greater risk, such as dentists, dental surgery assistants and hygienists, should be immunised as well as those travelling to high endemic hepatitis areas of the world. This involves three injections, the second 1 month and the third 6 months after the initial injection. Hence, adequate protection is not obtained until 6 months. Indeed, confirmation of protection after the third dose should be checked with serology for hepatitis B antibody. Over 95% are protected after three injections but a small number may require a fourth. It is also advisable that booster injections should be given every 5 years. However, immunisation does not eliminate the need for sensible precautions for avoiding the risk of infection from known carriers.

Specific hepatitis B immunoglobulin (HBIG) is available for use in association with the vaccine for laboratory or other personnel who have received 'needle stick' exposure to contaminated blood.

Dental care

As it is not possible or practical to screen all patients, it is therefore necessary to use a strict aseptic technique. The treatment of patients with acute hepatitis should be avoided until the patient has recovered.

In any patient with liver disease, the coagulation time should always be checked before any surgical procedures are undertaken. This is because the liver is responsible for the production of clotting factors, which may consequently be impaired.

Hepatitis C (HCV)

The existence of a further, probably virus-induced hepatitis, has been known for many years and by elimination it has been termed non-A, non-B hepatitis. Transmission seems to occur in a similar way to hepatitis B. In 1988 the identity of this RNA virus became known and it has now been termed hepatitis C. Prior to screening, it was believed that this virus was responsible for 90–95% of cases of post-transfusion hepatitis. Blood is now being screened in the UK for this virus to eliminate its potential spread, particularly as it is commonly responsible for the development of chronic active hepatitis.

There is a high risk of infection among haemophiliac patients, intravenous drug users, patients on haemodialysis, and possibly homosexuals. As transmission is similar to that of HBV, by exposure to blood, dentists may be at an increased risk.

Infectious mononucleosis (glandular fever)

This is caused by the Epstein–Barr virus and usually causes malaise, a sore throat, fever and cervical lymphadenopathy. Frank jaundice occurs in about 5% of patients, although mildly abnormal liver function tests may be seen in up to 25% of patients. Complete resolution of the hepatitis is usual without any sequelae.

15 Problems Related to the Prevention of Oral Disease

Dietary Related Disorders

There are many dietary related disorders, and these are generally classified as primary or secondary. Primary disorders are those which result from an inappropriate intake of food substances, and secondary disorders arise as a consequence of systemic, genetic or metabolic disturbances with dietary implications.

All chronically sick people need regular dental supervision, but certain medical conditions that affect the dietary intake may have a direct relationship to caries prevalence and may therefore require increased preventive care.

Primary disorders

Obesity

There is much that is still not known regarding obesity. It may be due simply to taking in more food than is required, thus there is an imbalance between calorific intake and expenditure.

In Western society, food has become more than just a nutritional intake, it is also a social factor and of considerable importance as a reward, motivator and token of affection. Many children are over-indulged, particularly those who have a handicap or chronic medical condition, as a means of compensation for their disability. They may become obese, which may further add to their impairment. It is particularly important that those people confined to a wheelchair do not become overweight and thus make life more difficult for themselves and their carers.

Although excessive calorific intake is overwhelmingly the most important cause of obesity it is not quite such a simple explanation. There are also other contributory causes, for example, hypothalamic disease, such as Prader–Willi syndrome (*see* page 68), endocrinopathies, such as hypothyroidism (*see* pages 58,59), Cushing's syndrome(*see* page 56) and Down's syndrome (*see* pages 65–67).

Excessive obesity may result in cardiovascular and respiratory disorders and the patient may be at risk with a general anaesthetic.

Anorexia nervosa and bulimia nervosa

These conditions are chronic psychosomatic illnesses manifested as eating disorders. They most commonly affect adolescent females. There is undernutrition and weight loss as a result of an obsession to be slim. Symptoms include depression, insomnia and a sensitivity to cold. Amenorrhoea occurs quite early in the condition, the heart is slow (bradycardia) and the blood pressure low (hypotension). Bulimia nervosa is characterised by marked overeating or 'binges' which are followed by self-induced vomiting and purging with laxatives.

Medical management

Treatment is initially aimed at restoring the body weight which may require hospitalisation. There is no consensus of opinion as to the most successful management for these patients either a cognitive or behavioral approach with self monitoring and positive reinforcement to start eating sensibly through dietary education, or psychiatric treatment in association with antidepressants. Both have their successes and failures.

The caries present in these patients may be accounted for by an analysis of their diet, which reveals frequent intakes of fermentable carbohydrate snacks as well as frequent drinks of fruit squashes and juices which are taken to quench the thirst of dehydration resulting from vomiting. The patients may be reluctant to admit to inducing vomiting. Evidence of erosion on the palatal aspects of the upper anterior teeth and the palatal aspects of the posterior teeth should arouse suspicion (perimylolysis) (*see* page 115). Dentists may therefore play an important role by detecting anorexia and bulimia nervosa and refer the patient for appropriate help.

Dietary habits

108

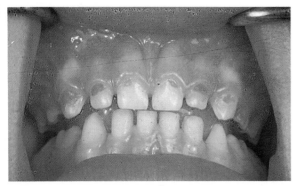

108 Caries affecting the labial aspect of the primary upper incisors and canines in a 3-year-old who was still having a bottle containing milk and sugar at bedtime.

Sick young children may be given sweet substances by overindulgent parents, relatives and friends or they may have a 'comforter' bottle containing a sweetened drink. This 'bottle caries' has a characteristic distribution initially affecting the labial surfaces of the maxillary incisors and the occlusal surfaces of the first primary molars (**108**). This pattern of caries is related to the sequence of eruption, duration of nursing and the position of the tongue, cheeks and lips during suckling. If the bottle is taken to bed, the caries process is considerably increased as a result of the reduced salivary flow and buffering capacity that occurs during the night.

Elderly people are also particularly at risk of developing caries. The cervical regions of the teeth are affected resulting in root caries. This is due to a combination of factors: exposure of cementum on the root surfaces as a result of gingival recession, possible reduction in the salivary flow with a change in its composition, a deterioration in oral hygiene standards and a reliance on sugar-containing convenience foods.

Secondary disorders

Secondary dietary related disorders occur in conditions which involve dietary control as part of their management.

Carbohydrate metabolism

There are several disorders of carbohydrate metabolism which require dietary restrictions. The most common of these is diabetes mellitus (*see* pages 51–53). Treatment involves the administration of insulin in insulin-dependent diabetes mellitus (IDDM) and a low carbohydrate diet with restriction of sucrose. Some early studies indicated that diabetic people showed an increased incidence of dental caries possibly due to an increase in the salivary sugar. More recent studies have suggested that young diabetic children at the onset of the disease exhibit a higher carious activity than a control group of healthy children. However, when the condition was stabilised, the dietary restrictions led to a decrease in dental caries.

Phenylketonuria

A strict diet is essential in phenylketonuria (PKU) following the diagnosis within the first few days of life (*see* page 54). If this diet, which must be low in phenylalanine and high in carbohydrate, is not followed severe intellectual impairment will occur. The carbohydrate portion of the diet provides 62% of the total calories required. In addition to the main meals, sucrose-containing snacks and drinks are encouraged. This diet therefore contains twice as much sugar as recommended diets for the normal child. The high and frequent intake of sucrose might be expected to promote a high incidence of carious lesions. However, the caries experience in the permanent dentition of children with PKU does not appear to be different from that found in those examined in national UK surveys. It has been suggested that further investigation is required into the possible protective effects of low phenylalanine diets.

Cystic fibrosis

People with cystic fibrosis require a diet which is high in calories and protein (*see* page 39). Steatorrhaea is a problem because of the lack of pancreatic enzymes; however, in order to increase the caloric density it is advisable to raise the fat content of the diet. The administration of a gastric secretor inhibitor before meals has proved effective in reducing the steatorrhaea. Pancreatic extracts are also necessary: previously these had to be sprinkled on the food and were unpleasant to taste and smell, but they are now in a more acceptable form as enteric coated granules.

The diet for people with cystic fibrosis, as that for those with PKU might suggest a high caries risk, but epidemiological evidence suggests the reverse. It is clear that our knowledge of caries is far from complete. The low caries rate may be linked to the frequent intake of antibiotics and the pancreatic extracts. The increased salivary pH and buffering capacity may also play a part, along with the increased levels of calcium and phosphates. The high calcium and phosphate content of the saliva may additionally contribute to the increase in calculus formation that is commonly seen in people with cystic fibrosis.

Chronic renal failure

The suggested diet for people with chronic renal failure is a low protein and low potassium content with supplementary carbohydrates (*see* pages 42,43). These carbohydrates are often given in a sugary form, as with children with cystic fibrosis. An increase in the caries incidence in children with renal disease has been reported and consequently frequent examinations and increased preventive measures are essential for these patients.

Coeliac disease

Gluten must be excluded from the diet as even small amounts may cause a relapse in the condition (*see* page 61). As gluten is widely used in convenience foods, soups, flavoured crisps etc., it is essential that all foods are carefully checked as to their contents. Preparation of a gluten-free diet is time consuming.

If gluten is ingested there may be malabsorption of vitamin D and calcium, which in the child may result in hypoplastic enamel defects in those teeth calcifying at that time.

Medication and Caries

There is now incontrovertible evidence, from epidemiological, clinical, animal and laboratory studies, linking sugar with dental caries. Not only is sugar a very large component of the normal Western diet, but as already stated, it is a much higher component in certain dietary related disorders. In addition, children who require medication over a long period or at frequent intervals may be receiving more sucrose as a result of the medicines prescribed. Many paediatric medicines are formulated in a sugar base. This has several advantages, including masking the taste of the drug, and acting as a preservative, an antioxidant and as a bulking agent.

There has been accumulating evidence since the 1950s that the sugar in medication taken over a prolonged period of time, might be a potential dental problem (**109**). The most conclusive evidence emerged in 1979, with the first epidemiological study into the relationship between medicines and dental caries. Children who were on long-term sucrose-based medicines had almost 3 times as many decayed, missing and filled teeth as a control group. Since then there has been further confirmation in other studies and it is now known that the problem is not confined to children.

Caries has also been reported with tablet preparations containing sucrose which are recommended to be chewed.

There is evidence to show that those with chronic medical disorders requiring long-term medication are at risk of contracting caries as a consequence of their treatment. In some patients, notably those with blood dyscrasias and cardiac, renal, metabolic and immuno-deficiency disorders, it is possible that dental disease, infection or treatment procedures may jeopardise their health or even their life.

Patients with poor muscular control, such as those with cerebral palsy, retain substances in their mouths for prolonged periods, thus medicines, especially those with a syrupy consistency are kept in contact with the teeth for a longer time. The cariogenic effect is increased when the medicines are taken at night, a time when the salivary flow and buffering capacity are reduced.

Not only are the consequences of dental disease greater in the medically compromised patient but there may also be considerable problems in carrying out the dental treatment. It has been shown that handicapped children receive significantly less restorative treatment and more extractions than normal children. These procedures may only be possible under a general anaesthetic with its additional morbidity.

As a result of the accumulating evidence associating sucrose-based medication with the development of dental caries, strenuous efforts have been made by the pharmaceutical industry to formulate medicines without sucrose. It is essential, that whenever, possible sugar-free medicines should be prescribed and if these are not available, there should then be special emphasis on preventive care.

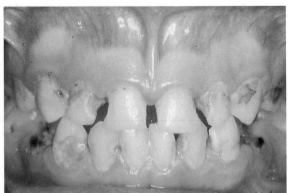

109 This patient suffers from epilepsy and has been taking sucrose based medication. He has developed rampant caries – that is caries proceeding at a rapid rate and affecting those areas of the teeth which are not normally susceptible.

Erosion of the Dental Tissues

Epidemiological data on the incidence of dental erosion are scanty, but clinical observation suggests that although this is not a widespread condition, it is a significant problem in a few people. The erosive effects on enamel of the excessive intake of fruit drinks and other acidic beverages is now well known. There has been an enormous increase in the sales of soft drinks over the past 10 years and it is likely that the incidence of erosion will increase.

Gastro-oesophageal reflux is also an important aetiological factor and should be investigated if suspected. In childhood, this reflux is quite common but is a cause for concern when it occurs over a long period of time. It may be associated with feeding difficulties, oesophagitis, anaemia and oesophageal stricture formation. There may be recurrent pneumonia secondary to aspiration. Early recognition of this disorder in handicapped children is of paramount importance in order that associated problems, including dental erosion, may be prevented.

The association between mentally handicapped people and gastro-oesophageal reflux was made in 1957, although the aetiology remains unknown. Several possible contributory factors mentioned have been extension spasms, incoordination of deglutition, kyphosis, scoliosis and prolonged recumbency; all of these factors may be present in people with cerebral palsy.

Gastro-oesophagheal reflux also occurs in those with

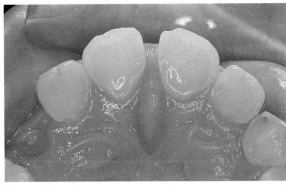

110

110 Erosion of the palatal aspect of the upper permanent incisor teeth associated with gastro-oesophageal reflux.

anorexia nervosa, and bulimia nervosa related to the self-induced vomiting.

Erosion (perimylolysis) is usually seen first on the palatal aspects of the maxillary incisor teeth (**110**), although the palatal and lingual aspects of premolar and molar teeth may all become affected. This may result in sensitivity and if the erosion is severe there may be exposure of the pulps.

The three factors in tooth tissue loss are erosion, attrition and abrasion, and they always occur in combination, but where erosion is the major factor certain preventive measures may be taken.

Medical management

Reflux oesophagitis may be controlled either by an alginate which forms a foaming agent on the gastric contents, or metoclopramide hydrochloride which improves oesophageal motility and sphincter function, or thirdly an H_2 receptor antagonist, e.g. cimetidine or ranitidine, or finally a proton pump inhibitor

omeprazole.

Some alginate tablets contain glucose and sucrose and instructions 'to be chewed after meals and at bedtime' may result in rampant caries. Infant forms are now available as a sugar-free powder.

Dental treatment

This should be directed towards preventing further erosion and eliminating pain.

Study casts should be made for accurate monitoring of on-going tooth tissue loss. A vacuum-formed splint filled with magnesium hydroxide or sodium bicarbonate may be of value if worn during danger periods to help

neutralise the acidic effects of the reflux activity. This procedure may not be tolerated by mentally handicapped patients. Exposed dentine should be covered if possible by one of the glass ionomer cements or dentine bonding agents.

Preventive Therapy

It cannot be stressed enough that prevention of dental disease is vitally important for people with health impairments, because life threatening complications may develop as a result of oral problems. Although prevention is important for everyone, there are people with specific conditions which have already been referred to for whom a full range of preventive measures should be provided (**111**).

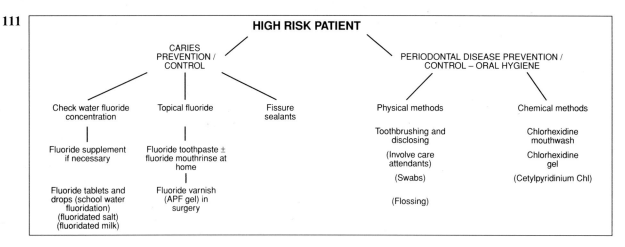

111 Preventive strategies for the high risk patient.

Prevention and control of dental caries

Dietary control

The most important aspect of prevention of caries is by a common sense approach to diet, and close liaison with dieticians is beneficial. The basis for dietary control is the restriction to meal times of foods containing fermentable carbohydrates, drinks containing sugar, and sugar-based medicines.

Most dentitions are not adversely affected by 3–4 sugary 'insults' a day although some are more susceptible than others. Following the intake of food or drinks containing sucrose there is a lowering of the pH. The critical pH of 5.5, when demineralisation of enamel begins, is reached within 2 minutes and returns to resting level in approximately 30 minutes. The increasing frequency with which sucrose is ingested prolongs the time that the critical pH is exceeded, allowing demineralisation to take place.

Frequency of consumption of sucrose is almost always related to total consumption and advice should be given to limit both the frequency and the amount of foods and drinks containing sucrose.

There are obviously some dietary related disorders that make such advice difficult to comply with. In these circumstances consultation with the dietitian is essential. Another aspect that may need to be taken into consideration is the time at which food, drink and particularly medication are taken. There is a circadian rhythm to salivary flow with a marked reduction in flow and buffering capacity at night. It is therefore more harmful to eat or drink fermentable carbohydrates immediately before going to bed or during the night.

Fluorides

Undoubtedly, the cornerstone of any community based caries preventive programme should be fluoridation of the drinking water.

The surveys that have been carried out into the dental condition of people with handicapping problems and impaired health have shown the considerable benefits of water fluoridation. These are even more cost effective than for the 'normal' population. However, where fluoridation is not possible, attention must be given to alternative sources of supplementary fluoride. Fluoride tablets and drops are suggested as the main sources of supplementation in the UK and USA, but there is increasing use of fluoridated salt and milk in Europe.

Fluoride tablets and drops should be recommended for all children who do not live in an optimally fluoridated area and who are medically compromised or handicapped in any way. There has been some controversy regarding the dosage because of reports of mottled enamel associated with supplementary fluorides.

This has become noticeable with the almost universal use of toothpaste containing fluoride in developed countries. It has been shown that under the age of 3 years almost half the toothpaste used is swallowed and in 3–4 year-olds approximately a third is ingested.

The dosages of fluorides which are currently suggested are shown in Table 1. Advice should be given that in order to achieve a topical effect as well as a systemic effect, the tablets should be sucked and not just swallowed.

Table 1. Dosages of supplementary fluorides to be given to medically compromised or handicapped children.

	Water fluoridation concentration	
	< 0.3 ppm	0.3–0.7 ppm
Age	**Dosage**	
6–24 months	0.25mg	—
2–4 years	0.5mg	0.25mg
Over 4 years	1.0mg	0.5mg

The major problem with supplementary fluorides is the compliance with a daily regimen. However, if the benefit of up to a 50% reduction is explained to the parents of 'at risk' children, then motivation has been found to be higher than for the general population.

Topical fluorides can be broadly divided into those used at home and those administered in the surgery. The division of fluorides into systemic and topical is an arbitrary one, water fluoridation and supplementary fluorides also have a topical effect. Conversely, as previously described, there may be a considerable amount of toothpaste ingested in the young patient. Fluoride toothpastes are obviously a very important preventive measure and should be advocated for all children. There are now available specially formulated junior or children's toothpastes, the majority containing 500 ppm fluoride and instruction should be given to use only a pea-sized amount.

Fluorides available that can be applied topically in the surgery include acidulated phosphate fluoride (APF) gels, stannous and sodium fluoride solutions, and fluoride varnishes. Extensive research has shown that there are significant benefits in caries control. The APF gels have to be applied in trays for 4 minutes with good moisture control, whereas the varnish contains a hydrophilic lacquer and is less sensitive to moisture contamination. The time involved, and patient compliance, usually make the varnish the method of choice. However, the varnish contains over 22,000 ppm fluoride compared with 12,300 ppm in APF gels, and care must be taken to avoid acute fluoride toxicity by using only small amounts. The topical fluoride application is necessary 2–3 times a year (*see* specialised text).

Fluoride mouth rinses can be very effective, particularly in controlling the rampant and root caries that may develop following radiotherapy and certain drug therapies. The daily use of a 0.05% neutral sodium fluoride solution has been shown to be the most effective. There are a number of proprietary brands available. Children under the age of 6 years, those with cerebral palsy and many intellectually impaired people may be unable to rinse and spit out adequately. It is, therefore, wise to check on this before prescribing any mouthrinse.

Fissure sealants

All children whose health is impaired, or who are physically or mentally handicapped, should be considered priority groups for the placing of fissure sealants. Other priority groups are those children who have had a high caries experience in the past and socially disadvantaged children.

It has been shown that the combination of water fluoridation and fissure sealants prevents almost 90% of caries.

The first and second permanent molar teeth are the most at risk from fissure caries but pits and fissures in the premolar teeth and pits on the palatal aspect of the upper permanent incisors may also require sealants. It has been stated that if a tooth has not become carious within 5 years of eruption then it is unlikely to be affected. However, recent studies have shown that this susceptible period seems to be increasing. The earlier a tooth can be fissure sealed after eruption the better. Unfortunately the technique is extremely moisture sensitive and a dry field is absolutely essential if the sealant is to be retained. There may, therefore, be practical difficulties in placing fissure sealants in some children where co-operation cannot be achieved.

Prevention and control of periodontal disease
Toothbrushing

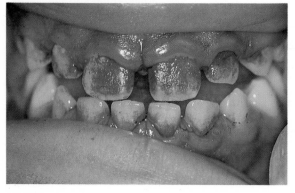

In general the techniques for toothbrushing for a compromised person are the same as those for anyone else. The most natural brushing methods are the horizontal scrub, a rotary motion, or simply an up-and-down movement. If toothbrushing is effective there is no need to alter the method. Even with a severe physical handicap it may be possible to achieve a high standard of oral hygiene (**112**).

The use of disclosing solutions is helpful in showing patients any problem areas (**113,114**).

112 Man with phocomelia as a result of his mother taking thalidomide during pregnancy. He achieves a satisfactory level of oral hygiene by holding his toothbrush between his toes.

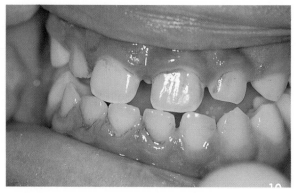

113 The mouth of this mentally handicapped girl has been disclosed.

114 The level of oral hygiene cleansing the girl in **113** was able to achieve unaided.

No one toothbrush design is suitable for all patients, however, a toothbrush with a flat surface head and round-ended multi-tufts is probably best. The design of the handle is of importance and adaptations may be helpful to increase the size for an easier grip. This may be achieved with a custom-made acrylic grip, a bicycle handle-bar grip, a ball or polystyrene tube (**70**). For patients with neuromuscular weakness, handles may be modified with a lightweight material such as foam. For patients unable to grasp the handle, the attachment of an elastic cuff or strap may be helpful. The handles of some toothbrushes can be bent to a more suitable angle.

Electric toothbrushes, although not a panacea for all oral hygiene problems, may be especially useful if the patient is able to place the toothbrush in the mouth but does not have the manual dexterity necessary to brush the teeth. They are heavier than a conventional toothbrush and there may be difficulties with the on/off switch.

Some carers feel happier using an electric toothbrush rather than a conventional one.

Totally effective plaque removal cannot be achieved by toothbrushing alone, but also requires some interproximal cleansing. Flossing is difficult to achieve for many able-bodied people and many lack the dexterity or the motivation necessary. Flossing or the use of wood points or interdental brushes should only be introduced on a selective basis to those who have mastered toothbrushing.

In some severely mentally handicapped people cleansing, may be facilitated by using a cloth, particularly to remove debris from the buccal sulcus (**115**).

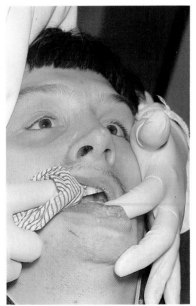

115 Demonstrating a method of cleaning the teeth with a cloth in a severely disturbed, mentally handicapped young man.

Chemical plaque control

The removal of plaque by physical means may be impossible for some people with physical or mental handicaps. Extensive research has produced some chemical anti-plaque agents, the most effective at the present time is chlorhexidine gluconate. This prevents a build-up of plaque as well as reducing the plaque that has accumulated in the absence of brushing. The chlorhexidine is absorbed to the hard and soft tissues in the target area, then released slowly in an active form.

The optimum concentration of chlorhexidine in a mouthwash is 0.12%, but there are several side effects at this level. Unfortunately, it has a rather unpalatable taste, even when masked by a mint flavouring, and it affects the taste sensation. It also causes extrinsic staining of the teeth which can be minimised by toothbrushing with an ordinary toothpaste and by regular prophylaxis by the dentist or hygienist. If mouth rinsing is not possible, chlorhexidine may be used in a gel form or applied by swabs or cotton buds. The gel form is not as effective an anti-plaque agent as is the mouthrinse but may be easier to use in children and mentally handicapped people.

There are now many commercially available anti-plaque and anti-calculus mouth rinses, but as yet, none of them replace the effectiveness of physical plaque removal by toothbrushing.

Involvement of the carer

They are many compromised children and adults who are unable to carry out oral hygiene procedures by themselves. It is not just the physical ability that is required but also the necessary motivation. It is essential that all those involved in their care are instructed in how to maintain their oral health. Some carers find an electric tooth brush more acceptable to use.

If help is required in toothbrushing, the position of the carer is important. One helpful position is for the carer to stand behind the patient who is seated in a straight-backed chair or their wheelchair. The carer can then stabilise the patient's head against them by cradling it in one arm against his or her body, leaving the other arm free for brushing. Another position that may be helpful is to have the patient supine on the floor or settee with his or her head supported in the carer's lap.

The maintenance of the dentition is even more important in patients with severe physical disabilities who are able to achieve a measure of independence by using their mouth as an accessory limb. A mouthpiece can be constructed with special 'mouth sticks' that can be adapted to operate a word processor, turn pages in a book, etc. (**116–118**).

116

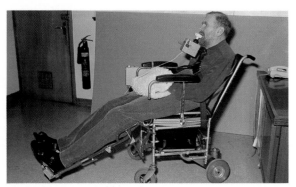

116 Patient who has multiple sclerosis and is able to move only his head.

117

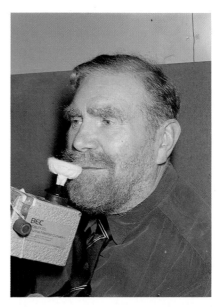

117 Modification to wheelchair motor controls to enable the patient some independence by manoeuvring his own wheelchair with his mouth.

118

118 Intra-oral view of the patient shown in **115**. Maintenance of the health of his dentition by the dentist, hygienists and his carers is vital in order for him to continue some degree of independence.

Drug Induced Gingival Hyperplasia

Phenytoin

The effect that phenytoin has on the gingival tissue has been known for some time This drug is used very successfully in the control of epilepsy and has minimal side effects. However, in about 50% of patients collagen production and fibroblastic activity are affected, resulting in gingival hyperplasia (**76**). In some patients this is minimised if there is good oral hygiene (**74,75**). Surgical removal of the hyperplastic tissue may be necessary to improve the aesthetics and periodontal condition, but there may be recurrence if the drug is not changed and the oral hygiene is not maintained at a very high level. However, the patient's physician should be consulted – if a patient is well controlled, it may not be considered advisable to alter his or her therapy.

Prophylaxis and maintenance of good oral hygiene will help to minimise gingival problems. Chlorhexidine mouthwashes have also been shown to be beneficial.

Cyclosporin

Many transplant units are now using a combination of azathioprine, prednisolone and cyclosporin, each in a low dose, to prevent graft rejection and reduce the likelihood of dose-related side effects. One of the side effects is gingival hypertrophy. This appears clinically different from that caused by phenytoin and is at present undergoing research.

Nifedipine

Gingival enlargement has been reported with calcium channel blocking drugs and nifedipine is the drug most frequently implicated, perhaps because it is the one most commonly prescribed in the treatment of angina and hypertension (*see* page 24). About 10% of patients on this drug develop gingival hyperplasia but the aetiology remains uncertain but is thought to be due to high levels of nifedipine in the plasma. It resembles phenytoin gingival hyperplasia both clinically and histologically. Improved oral hygiene may achieve some reduction in the hyperplasia. Surgical removal of excessive tissue may be necessary but the patient should be warned that it may recur. The maintenance of good oral hygiene is essential.

Self Mutilation

Unfortunately, the teeth can also be used as destructive agents as well as for incising and masticating food. Some people with severe mental handicap may become very frustrated and may resort to mutilation either of themselves or their carers. Usually the hands or fingers are chewed resulting in excoriated keratotic lesions (**119**). There are two specific syndromes which are associated with self mutilation, Lesch–Nyhan syndrome and congenital insensitivity to pain.

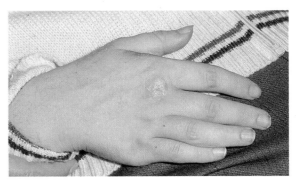

119

119 Self mutilation of the hands, showing excoriated keratotic lesions.

Lesch–Nyhan syndrome

This is a rare congenital disorder of purine metabolism and is associated with athetosis, hyperuricaemia and mental and physical retardation; it usually occurs in boys. There is an overwhelming desire to bite any part of the anatomy which is accessible, particularly the lips and fingers. The destruction may be so severe that in order to prevent further damage the teeth may have to be extracted, a decision which requires consultation with the parents or guardians and the consultant medical supervisor.

Congenital insensitivity to pain

This is also a rare condition with uncertain aetiology, in which self mutilation is accidental rather than deliberate. Burns are common occurrences and even fractures may occur without the person being aware of them. Normally the resulting pain causes immediate removal from an intense source of heat but those with insensitivity do not retract and are thus further damaged (**120,121**).

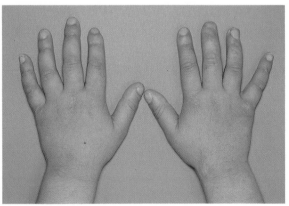

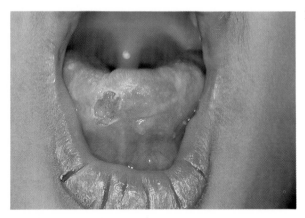

120 Damaged fingertips in a child with congenital insensitivity to pain as a result of holding his fingers against a very hot radiator.

121 Self inflicted trauma to the tongue and lips in a patient with congenital insensitivity to pain.

Gingivitis artefacta

This should be considered in patients with unusual gingival lesions with no apparent aetiology. It is due to habitual picking by the fingers of the oral mucosa, usually the gingivae (**122**). It occurs in two peaks: in 3–6-year-olds and in adolescence. In the young child it may start as an itching sensation in the gum at the time of tooth eruption and become a habit (**123**). Usually all that is required is to show the lesion to both the child and their parent and advise cessation of the habit, and this generally results in resolution. In the adolescent it may be an attention seeking device, advice should be given but occasionally psychiatric help may be necessary to find out the underlying reason for this self mutilation.

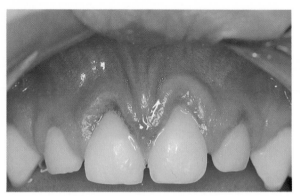

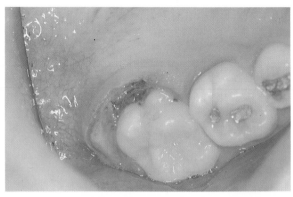

122 Gingival recession around the primary incisor teeth in a 3-year-old as a result of habitual picking of the gum with a finger nail (gingivitis artefacta).

123 Gingival inflammation on the palatal aspect of the maxillary first permanent molar in a 6-year-old child (gingivitis artefacta).

Bibliography

Baraitser, M. and Winter, R. (1988) *A Colour Atlas of Clinical Genetics,* Wolfe Publishing Ltd.

Behrman, R.E. and Vaughan, V.C. (1987) *Nelson Textbook of Paediatrics*, W.B. Saunders Co.

Berkow, R. and Fletcher, A.J. (Eds.) (1987) *The Merck Manual,* Merck, Sharp and Dohme Research Laboratories.

Gorlin, R.J., Cohen, M.M. and Levin, L.S. (1990) *Syndromes of the Head and Neck*, 3rd Edition, Oxford University Press.

Gorlin, R.J. and Goldman, H.M. (Eds.) (1970) *Thoma's Oral Pathology ,* C.V. Mosby.

Kerr, D.A., Ash, M.M. and Millard, H.D. (1983) *Oral Diagnosis,* 6th Edition, C.V. Mosby.

Little, J.W. and Falace, D.A. (1980) *The Dental Management of the Medically Compromised Patient,* C.V. Mosby.

Lynch, M.A. (Ed.) (1977) *Burket's Oral Medicine Diagnosis and Treatment,* 7th Edition, J.B. Lippincott.

Murray, J.J., Rugg Gunn, A.J. and Jenkins, G.N. (1991) *Fluorides in Dental Caries Prevention,* 3rd Edition, Wright.

Neville,B.W., Damm, D.D., White, D.K. and Waldron, C.A. (1991) *A Colour Atlas of Clinical Oral Pathology,* Lea and Febiger.

Rowe, A.H.R. and Alexander, A.G. (Eds.) (1988) *Clinical Methods, Medicine, Pathology and Pharmacology,* Blackwell Scientific Publications.

Weatherall, D.J., Ledingham, J.G.G. and Warrell, D.A. (Eds.) (1990) *Oxford Textbook of Medicine,* 2nd Edition, Oxford University Press.

Wiedemann, H.R. Grosse, K.R. and Dibbern, H. (1986) *An Atlas of Characteristic Syndromes, A Visual Aid to Diagnosis,* Wolfe Publishing Ltd.

Index